Rosemary Conley was born in Leicester in 1946. She founded her own slimming club in 1973 and is now Managing Director of Successful Slimming Clubs. She has one daughter.

Successful Slimming Clubs is a Trade Name of IPC Magazines Ltd.

Also in Arrow by Rosemary Conley

EAT YOURSELF SLIM

EAT AND STAY SLIM

Rosemary Conley

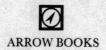

ARROW BOOKS

Arrow Books Limited
17–21 Conway Street, London W1P 6JD

An imprint of the Hutchinson Publishing Group

London Melbourne Sydney Auckland
Johannesburg and agencies throughout
the world

First published by Arrow 1985

© IPC Magazines Ltd 1985

Set in Linotron Baskerville

Photoset by Rowland Phototypesetting Ltd
Printed and bound in Great Britain
by Anchor Brendon Ltd,
Tiptree, Essex

ISBN 0 09 935820 4

To Michael with love

With grateful thanks to Tim Lacey of
Keith Hall Salons for the notes on hair
care, and to John Duggan for help with
exercise physiology.

Contents

Introduction

We know how to lose weight. It is *maintaining* our slimming success that is much more difficult. It *can* be done easily and permanently with the advice offered in this book. I will show you how to forget your bathroom scales, forget counting calories, and forget the paranoia developed from long-term dieting. There will be no more binges, no more gimmicks or crash diets. You will be able to eat normally again, and enjoy a wonderfully contented and healthy life! I will also help you to improve your sex life, attain a beautiful figure and at the same time make the most of yourself. I'll help you put back the confidence often lost while overweight. You won't believe the new you that can emerge.

When I started my first slimming club in 1973 after fighting my own overweight battle, I adopted a completely new dieting concept, proved by myself and a few friends who volunteered to help. My philosophy actually proved that you could lose weight on a generous calorie intake and consequently achieve weight maintenance thereafter.

This was a far cry from the ideas promoted by the medical profession. Most diet advisers at that time were recommending their overweight patients (or members if they attended a slimming club) to eat the bare minimum of food, usually around 1,000 calories per day. This resulted in enormous frustration for the slimmers because they were continually hungry. If they persevered and actually lost their surplus weight on such a small intake, their metabolic rate had inevitably reduced considerably, which resulted in them regaining all the lost weight in no time without actually overeating! Often they panicked and began binge eating, which then resulted in them actually weighing *more* at the end than they were in the beginning.

Our metabolic rate adjusts according to an increase or decrease in the consumption of calories and expending of energy. In other words a large reduction in calorie intake reduces metabolic rate significantly, whilst a small reduction in calorie intake reduces metabolic rate only very slightly.

Exercise taken regularly *increases* the metabolic rate. It therefore stands to reason that if you make a small reduction in calories it will only have a slight effect on your metabolic rate, while an increase in physical activity will effectively increase it. Consequently if you can diet on an increased calorie intake that still effects a satisfactory weight loss (usually between 1,400 and 1,600 calories per day) and at the same time increase your physical activity, you will lose your unwanted weight quickly and maintain your metabolic rate throughout. If you participate in a good deal of exercise, you could even increase it while you are dieting! This in itself is wonderful, but more important is the fact that you can maintain your slimmer figure with virtually no chance of regaining your weight, unless, of course, you grossly overeat. One of the most gratifying statements I hear from members who have lost many stones is their announcement to the class: 'I'm now eating normally again and I thought I would have to diet for the rest of my life.'

By 1980 my original slimming clubs (called Slimming and Good Grooming) had blossomed to fifty weekly classes in my home town of Leicester. I had a total membership of around 20,000 and I knew by then that my philosophy really did work. I had thousands upon thousands of successful slimmers to prove it.

Later that year I was approached by IPC Magazines Ltd, who publish some of the most popular women's magazines in the country – *Woman, Woman's Own, Woman's*

Realm, Woman & Home, etc. IPC had their own *Successful Slimming* magazine and they felt that a slimming club was the obvious way to broaden their horizons. It was all very exciting when they asked me to organise it on their behalf, and six months later I sold SAGG Ltd to them. Here I am in 1985 still loving every minute of my job as Managing Director of Successful Slimming Clubs. My terrific staff at our head office in Leicester, and the exceptional capabilities of my managers and lecturers, have enabled the clubs to increase to many hundreds, and our total membership now stands at around 130,000.

Over the years my philosophy has been gradually adopted by the medical profession, and even by other slimming clubs as they realised they were causing problems rather than solving them by recommending 'starvation'-type diets! (My first book *Eat Yourself Slim* explains this philosophy in detail.)

'That's fine,' I hear you say, 'but I was one of those who starved herself slim – what hope have I got?' Within *Eat and Stay Slim* I give careful instructions on how to effectively increase your metabolic rate and ultimately eat normally again without worrying about increasing your weight. It really can be done, but it will take a little time and some patience. What a small price to pay for a passport to successful weight maintenance for ever.

Several products are mentioned within this book. I can assure readers that all references or recommendations are made only after personally using these products. I hope you will use this book as a friend. After getting to know it I hope you will refer to it regularly to read again the advice that will help you to live life to the full.

1
Feeling great with the new you!

At last you have made it. There you are one morning preening yourself in front of the mirror. Yes the same one you have avoided for a long time. Tummy – just visible. Weight – fine. Hips – narrower. You are, and with full justification, bright-eyed and bushy-tailed that day, and very happy. You have finally made your goal weight; something you have worked very hard at for weeks, or maybe even months. The world is, indeed, a rosy place. So why should I come along at this very satisfying time to issue words of warning? Well, as mother used to say when giving you a dose of medicine, because it's good for you.

For a start you can discard your bathroom scales – that is my way of making sure you realise the full implication of what you have just achieved. This will also emphasise that there should be no going back along the road down which you have just struggled. After all, what a waste of time, energy and money to go back to where you started; yet thousands of people do. The various reasons for their downfall will be discussed in later chapters because I believe if you understand them, you are halfway to winning the battle.

There is no easy way to slim, but it can be done and you've just done it. I've done it too, and so have thousands of members of my Successful Slimming Clubs. But my experience of running these clubs all over the country has taught me one fundamental lesson: taking off the weight is the easiest part, *keeping* it off is most definitely the hardest.

As I have already said, forget the scales, but let's move over to the mirror. Take a good look at yourself with your clothes on. Why dressed? Because that's how the majority of people see you, and because we can all find 'an inch to pinch' if we look at ourselves naked, and often we can be too critical about our body.

Having taken a good look at yourself dressed give yourself another pat on the back for what you have achieved so far. If you find that difficult, try to wave the magic wand and cast your mind back to what you looked like when you first started your slimming campaign. See the difference? Of course you do, so now give yourself that well-earned praise. After all, you can go out today to buy that dress, skirt or pair of jeans you have dreamed about. Trying them on in the shop will be a real pleasure instead of causing you embarrassment. Rush home and show them to your husband, children or boyfriend and you will be amazed how good you feel, not to mention how proud they will be.

So why do so many people regain their lost weight?

For many people the reason is simply that they stay on their diet for much too long. They want to achieve a skinny figure which in most cases is completely unnatural to the body anyway. Remember, Twiggy did not have to diet to maintain her figure; she was born with it.

Secondly, as already briefly explained, our metabolic rate adjusts to however many calories our body is used to consuming. Metabolic rate is simply the rate at which we burn food, or our 'miles per gallon' if you prefer. But, unlike a car which uses a steady amount of fuel at a given speed consistently, our metabolic rate adjusts either up or down after we have been consuming a certain amount of calories. So, a person who has always had an enormous appetite will maintain his or her weight without fluctuation providing they continue to consume that amount. A dieter on the other hand will in time stop losing weight on a low intake no matter what it is – even 800 calories a day, which is ridiculously and dangerously low anyway. The slimmer would reach a plateau after a while despite the feeling of starvation!

What we have to realise is that we *can* INCREASE the

metabolic rate and allow ourselves to eat normally and so RETAIN our newly found slimmer body.

The increase in metabolic rate can be brought about in two ways: by slowly increasing the number of calories we consume each day, and also by increasing our activity level. You don't have to adopt both methods, but if you do there will, undoubtedly, be greater success. Anyone wanting to lose weight should do so by increasing their activity at the same time as moderately reducing their daily calorie intake. Doing this means that we are less likely to reach a plateau, which not only disheartens a dieter, but also forces her to further reduce her calorie intake resulting in a greater drop in her metabolic rate. It can become a vicious circle and one that must be avoided at all costs.

The successful dieter is the one who cuts down her food and steps up her quota of exercise. This is one of the main reasons why our Successful Slimming classes have such good results. We help members to lose weight by offering them a sensible and generous eating plan and providing Slimobility exercises. These are fun to do and certainly don't call for the same self-discipline required to go on an early morning jog or bike ride.

Many people believe that you cannot slim successfully unless you are young. One of my favourite members is a lady of sixty-three called Evelyn. She joined one of my classes eight years ago weighing in at a mammoth 15st 10lb (100 kilos). I say mammoth because Evelyn is only 5ft 2in, but she put her mind to become a successful slimmer and has maintained her new weight of between 8st 10lb and 9st 2lb (55 and 57 kilos) for more than five years. It was after losing 5 of her unwanted 7 stones that she asked me what she could do about her flabby, most unattractive chins. The stretching exercise I advised took only a few months of regular practice to achieve a total cure. Lean your head backwards, take your bottom teeth over your top lip and hold for a count of 3. Repeat 10 times.

17

The Slimobility classes we offer in conjunction with our slimming classes mean we are able to help members stay trim and attractive after they have achieved their goal weight. This not only allows them to keep a constant eye on their weight, but even more importantly, they become more confident with their newly found figure as they continue to attend the Slimobility classes. The exercises are themselves the reason for attending the classes.

Psychologically it would be wrong for someone to go to a slimming club just for a weight check. It is much more sensible to go for the exercises and then pop on the scales afterwards. It is so important to learn to relax about your weight and your new figure. *Remember you really won't wake up tomorrow having gained weight – not unless you overeat.*

One of the things that must be borne in mind when achieving a slimline figure after many years of being overweight is that considerable adjustments need to be made. You might be one of the lucky ones who can cope with the situation and naturally adopt the new role of the slimmer you. But it can sometimes create quite a problem learning to live with your new self. After all, you could feel a completely different person now. Certainly on the physical side there is nothing to compare with the previously flabby body which once surrounded you. Now that has gone, your genuine personality, hidden for so long behind that wall of flesh, can jump out and dazzle the world. Or can it?

You have to look on this as a rebirth, certainly on the physical side and almost as surely mentally too. In this book I do not intend to go into the deep psychology of slimming, but there are some tips I will pass on from my own experience and that of scores of others I have met at my classes over the years. Often the adjustment affects not only you, but also your family and friends, although I believe this is not so much a problem for the married woman because her husband has seen her reduce weight gradually and both have adapted to her new shape.

Many a marriage, however, has changed dramatically

as a result of the wife losing a significant amount of weight. It is strange how many husbands welcome a wife who is comparatively unattractive because he feels safe. An un-attractive wife is less likely to be approached by another male admirer – the husband is happy with the compan-ionship and friendship of his totally dependent and poss-ibly insecure wife. I have to say that many marriages have broken up because the wife suddenly realises that she has been used rather like a doormat for many years, and she had never realised her own qualities. I must hasten to add, however, that I'm sure many more marriages improve dramatically because the wife loses weight. For instance, Janet Gotch the winner of *Successful Slimming* magazine's Shape-Up Campaign in 1983 was one of our club mem-bers. Janet lost almost 6 stone and went from appearing to be a frumpy middle-aged woman to looking every bit a stunning 25-year-old. She now has a model-like figure and her husband, Joe, refers to her as his 'wonderful new wife'. Janet's weight loss has made an enormous difference to their marriage.

Evelyn, my lovely 63-year-old to whom I referred to earlier, is adored more than ever by her husband War-wick, although he loved her before she was slim. He beams with pride every time I see him with Evelyn, and I just know that she will never regain that weight which hung around her for all those years. They find it so amusing when they meet old friends from years ago who think Warwick has a new wife!

But take the woman who is going to meet a man for the first time who has never known her any other way but slim. Undoubtedly she will lack self-confidence; but she must learn to cope, otherwise life will lose many of the joys it could hold for her.

The answer must be to get out and about, meet people, go to parties, join organisations or groups. Nobody is pretending it is easy, particularly for those who are shy by nature – but remember that a few naturally slim girls are very unsure of themselves. Trying to be an extrovert after years of looking inwards is tough, but that does not mean it can't be done. I think it is a good idea to go into shops and try on lots of clothes. It doesn't matter if you don't intend to buy anything that day, just go in and talk to the assistant. Show yourself, listen to the compliments and enjoy it.

Start a sports campaign by buying a new swimsuit and take a regular dip in the local pool. The first time you step out of the changing room in your new bikini (or one-piece, if you prefer) you will want to turn and run back, quite forgetting that you are no longer the former large lady open to sniggers from rude and uncouth youths. Now you're an attractive woman, and the only glances you are going to get are admiring ones from those self-same tormentors.

You may still be a little self-critical of a slight figure imperfection because we are never going to think of ourselves as perfect, but don't let that worry you. The human race is by nature incredibly vain, and the comforting fact is that everybody else in that pool is far more conscious about *their* own appearance than they are about yours. As soon as you realise this the more confident you will feel about your own figure. It is very strange to realise that even somebody who is slimmer than you may look admiringly at your figure because you have, in her opinion, a slimmer waist or more slender thighs than she. We can very easily become far too self-critical, but one of the lessons that I hope to teach you is how to learn to like yourself and accept that admittedly there may be one or two areas which could be improved, but basically you are very fortunate to have the figure that you do.

One of the most difficult lessons to learn is how to cope with compliments. It is so easy when someone says how nice you look to brush it off and think they are being sarcastic or funny. Try to look at yourself and say 'I'm looking good, even quite attractive'. Let that confidence begin to emerge. It is a complimentary package or equation: Confidence equals attractiveness. You can *think* yourself into it. There is nothing more attractive than confidence itself. Learn to look people in the face, hold your head up high and walk tall. If you feel good believe me, you'll look good!

It is also important to realise that you don't need a 36–22–36 figure, a gorgeous face and waist-length hair to be attractive. If you wanted to be a film star or on the front cover of a women's magazine then such attributes would certainly help. There is, however, a limit to how many actresses are required for beautiful roles, and to be a top model you need to be tall and to have been born with a very slim figure. In fact such beauty can have its problems. A friend of mine knew a girl called Victoria who was incredibly beautiful with a stunning figure. One day my friend happened to raise the subject of what it must be like to be so perfect, to which Victoria responded: 'It's an absolute pain. No one wants to know the real me underneath; they're too busy letching at me or wanting to stroke my bottom! I can't find a real boyfriend – I only get invitations from men who want to drag me around with them like a top dog from Cruft's!'

It must be realised that you can still be considered very attractive without looking like a Greek goddess by making the most of your best assets. It may be that you have a sparkling personality or cause your friends to fall about laughing because of your tremendous sense of humour. Women can be considered attractive for all sorts of reasons, and often it is for qualities they didn't even realise they possessed until they are pointed out. So, don't prejudge yourself, but listen to compliments and realise where your strengths lie. Start learning to like yourself as you are and stop trying to be something you're not.

2
And now returning to normal eating

The key to maintaining a lower weight is simply eating sensible foods in moderate quantities. If you have lost weight on food which has been satisfying then it is easy to adjust, but if you have lost weight on starvation rations the adjustment requires more patience. However, there is no doubt it can be achieved just the same.

To enable us to determine the correct plan of action for readjustment we must first discover your current metabolic rate. It is possible to have your metabolic rate tested, and certain clinics offer this facility. However, it may be that such facilities are not within easy reach of your home and therefore we have to assess your metabolic rate by our own means. This is not difficult, but it requires just one week of very careful calorie counting, writing down absolutely everything you eat or drink – even that half sandwich that was left from the children's teatime! On page 23 you will see an example of a calorie record sheet. If you draw up a similar form on a fairly large piece of paper you can start the experiment. Before discarding the bathroom scales weigh yourself at the start of the test week, preferably first thing in the morning after going to the toilet, and ideally with no clothes on.

Please complete the following details prior to commencement of your diet this week:

Date.............. Weight today.............. Weight 7 days later..............

Measurements today:
Bust..............   Waist..............   Hips..............

After 7 days:
Bust..............   Waist..............   Hips..............

Diet Record Sheet

Please record absolutely everything that you eat this week. *Weigh* items, don't estimate quantities. Record every calorie, both for food and drinks. Don't be afraid of admitting to the occasional treats. You need to see *exactly* what you have consumed, as this is essential if you are to discover your current calorie intake/energy output ratio.

	Monday	Cals	Tuesday	Cals	Wednesday	Cals	Thursday	Cals	Friday	Cals	Saturday	Cals	Sunday	Cals
Breakfast														
Mid-morning														
Lunch														
Mid-Afternoon														
Evening Meal														
Supper														
Totals														

After careful monitoring of your total food and drink consumption during the following seven days, weigh yourself again and note your weight on the diet record sheet. IT IS IMPORTANT THAT YOU DO NOT ADD UP EACH DAY'S TOTAL CALORIES UNTIL AFTER YOU HAVE WEIGHED YOURSELF ON DAY SEVEN. DO NOT WEIGH YOURSELF IN BETWEEN. Ensure that conditions are as similar as possible to those at the beginning of your trial week; that is same time of day, same scales, naked, etc. During this trial week you should eat fairly normally, without obviously overeating or selecting particularly high-calorie foods. Ideally you should weigh your food and note the calorie values alongside *before* each meal.

The reason I say you must not add up each daily calorie total is because you may find you eat more 'because I haven't eaten many calories today', or you may even find that you abandon the exercise completely because you realise how much more you have eaten than usual and assume you will have gained loads of weight. I cannot emphasise enough the importance of learning to trust yourself and to get off the roundabout of worrying about what you've eaten, how many calories, what you are going to have next and so on. So after day 7 add up your calorie intake. After weighing yourself at the end of the seven-day period you will discover whether you have lost, gained or maintained weight on that calorie intake over a week. Whatever the result you will have a definite guide towards your current metabolic rate. If you have lost weight you can obviously increase your calorie intake and, in fact, should do so by about 200 calories per day. If your weight remained constant during the seven days try increasing your calories by 100 calories a day for a week in the hope of speeding up your metabolism, then add 100 a day for another week until you are confidently eating what you consider to be normal.

If there has been a weight gain then various questions must be asked. For instance is your menstrual period due?

Many women gain several pounds at this time because they retain fluid. However, some women experience no such increase at their period but at some other time during their menstrual cycle, at a regular time each month. Make a note in your diary to remind you at what part of the month your weight is affected. If there is no particular reason for gaining weight then there is obviously need for some action. First of all look at your calorie record sheet and see if you can spot where you particularly over-indulged. It may have been the day when you were unexpectedly taken out for a meal when you had already eaten a substantial lunch. It could have been the box of chocolates that your boyfriend gave you for your birthday. Your weight gain could be attributable to either of these events, and in future you should cut down after eating such an extravagance or alternatively ration yourself to having one or two chocolates per day. If there is no particular reason why you should have gained weight that week then check that you calculated your calorie values accurately. Then consider whether there are ways that you can cut down your calories without significantly altering your pattern of eating. Choose your food more carefully for the next week, selecting lower-calorie foods whenever possible. Also try to increase your activity level. This will certainly help to increase your metabolic rate and so prevent further weight gain. Obviously last week more calories were consumed than your body needed at that particular time. Don't despair, but give yourself a chance to get the balance of your calorie intake right. Try to be patient.

After discovering your current metabolic rate you will also know how much you can eat – even how much you can get away with. Soon confidence in this ability will grow and a more relaxed attitude will develop. I use the word 'relaxed' in a positive way; that you will have sufficient self-control to stop after a special treat and not despair after one failure. Every time you eat a treat and refrain from going off the rails completely into an eating binge, congratulate yourself. I cannot emphasise too strongly what a wonderful achievement it is each time you do this.

I know there are certain times when we feel helplessly out of control. Many women feel this just prior to a menstrual period. Even though I had a hysterectomy five years ago, around every twenty-eighth day I have an uncontrollable urge to overeat. I now quite look forward to it and I eat anything I want that day knowing that my desire to gorge will only last twenty-four hours. The following day I return to eating normally and the pound or two I gained quickly disappears. Having had such a good feast I don't feel so hungry over the next few days and the excess soon vanishes.

I used to find that on this one day in the month I was unbearable to live with; I lacked self-confidence and really hated myself for overeating. The next day I was so upset because I had failed yet again that I often used to have another binge. Life was one long battle of the binge and I had no idea where it would all end, which made me even more depressed! Now that I have discovered the reason for my bout of overeating I don't feel guilty about it, and strangely enough don't seem to eat so much. I am sure everyone has a reason for their binge problem and it is so important to find out what it is.

If you find yourself falling into a regular pattern of binge eating which you can't cope with, then maybe there is something fundamentally wrong with your life style. If it is your husband or family then do take the time to sit down and talk about it. One of the lessons I have learned in recent years is that often thoughts or worries at the back of my mind can blow up out of all proportion unless they are brought out into the open. So many problems could be avoided if they were only discussed between the parties concerned. I wonder how often you have allowed yourself to become upset only to find out at some later stage that in fact your unhappiness and concern were totally without foundation, and that you had just read the situation incorrectly. If you've got a problem, talk about it and sort it out. You'll be surprised how painless it is and what an enormous relief it will be to you to get it off your chest.

Maybe your problems stem from work, and it is often less easy to discuss things that are troubling you with your boss or your colleagues. For the last three years I have been in charge of a dozen or so female staff in the office and 300 slimming-club lecturers throughout the UK. It always disappoints me that despite the fact that I consider myself to be friendly and approachable, my staff are reluctant to discuss any problems with me. They presumably think I am far too busy to want to be bothered with what they assume I will consider unimportant issues. If only they realised that it would make my job considerably easier and their job infinitely more enjoyable if they did come to see me for a chat. There must be millions of employees and employers who feel exactly the same, and I can't help feeling that the same problems exist in a lot of marriages too!

If you know there is a problem in your life then it is worth attempting to discover the root cause. If you run away from it you'll be fighting against it for ever more. If you hate the work you do in your job then why not look for a new one. It may be that you would be happier serving in a shop than working in an office. Just because you've always worked in an office doesn't mean that it's the ideal job for you.

You may be capable of holding down a job that is quite different from anything you have ever tried before. It may be a type of employment which was out of reach before, but is quite within your capabilities now you are slim. There is no doubt that overweight employees are not as attractive to an employer as someone who is slimmer. Life can be even more exciting than you may realise, but you may need to help it happen. As we spend a major part of our life at work, it is vital that we are happy there. And of course, if we are really absorbed by our work food becomes less important. If we are bored in our work we tend to think of little else!

One of the most rewarding aspects of my job is that I see previously overweight ladies coming forward and training as Successful Slimming Club lecturers. They develop into confident and often stunningly attractive women who, a few years ago, would never have believed that they had it in them to stand in front of between 50 to 100 ladies, let alone convey such confidence to encourage them to shed their excess weight. Rather like a snake sheds its skin, the slimmer can shed that flabby fat and find beneath a beautiful firm body providing she goes about it in the right way. Sensible exercise not only firms the body, but it also helps to relax the mind.

The more you are able to change away from your old way of life the better. If you can change jobs it will be a great help in maintaining your new weight for all kinds of reasons. Your new colleagues will not try to 'fatten you up' like your previous ones may have done, particularly the plump ones! You can practise your new role to an audience who won't realise you're still learning the part! It will be so much fun!

If you are basically unhappy with your life style perhaps you should seriously consider making a change, whether it be your job, your home or even your companion! After all, if you are unhappy you will overeat again and regain all that lost weight, and then you'll be even more miserable. Face any problems you may have and sort them out now.

3
Getting out of the slimming habit

As we know, one of the main problems facing experienced slimmers is their paranoid attitude towards what they eat. They become obsessed with food and think of little else besides what they will have for the next meal, how many calories it contains and just how many foods are forbidden to them. If only they would realise that they can eat *anything* in moderation.

Another downfall is to continually weigh yourself. Sometimes slimmers weigh themselves several times a day in the hope of 'instant' results from avoiding food for half a day. Weight reduction shown on the scales is very misleading. When we consider that the majority of our body weight is fluid anyway, and for all kinds of reasons this can fluctuate from day to day, we must learn to leave weighing scales alone. A mirror and a waist belt will provide a much more accurate guide to fatness or slimness.

A mirror is even better than a best friend for making you realise if your weight is up or down. Although it can't speak, the reflection will be totally honest! The larger the mirror the better. I have two huge mirrors in my bedroom, and they certainly serve to remind me of my current size. Realising how you look and also learning to accept the imperfections is a vital step towards long-term success in weight maintenance.

A belt is a very accurate guide too. Those holes really don't move, so if the belt feels tighter, you've gained weight. Time to be careful before your weight gets out of hand. Don't diet, just moderate your eating for a day or two.

Unfortunately for some bored and overweight people, slimming can become a consuming hobby and scales their worst enemy. If they have little else to think about they regain their weight just to see the scales going up and down; there is a definite thrill in seeing that needle on the scales drop. They become yo-yo slimmers gaining weight just to see it go again. So put your scales well away in a tall cupboard or ask someone to hide them.

It is vital to find a formula of eating that suits you and your family. I have to admit to being the world's worst dieter. As soon as I become aware of calorie counting specific foods and restricting the quantities, I seem to want to eat more and more. So I have now discovered that the only way to maintain my weight, or to reduce it occasionally (after Christmas or a holiday), is to be very sensible about what I eat and also the quantities, without actually calorie counting. In other words I now have a natural instinct which tells me how far I can go.

Because the evenings are the most important time of the day for us, dinner always gets preferential treatment. It is always a large meal of meat or poultry with lots of vegetables. I always eat plenty of potatoes or rice and usually have a glass or two of wine. But I never eat a dessert if we are dining on our own.

Cutting out the sweet after the meal has really helped to curb my sweet tooth. Because of eating a substantial meal during the evening I am not too hungry at breakfast time, so I just eat fruit. For lunch in the office I have a jacket potato with cheese. I look forward to it all morning and enjoy every mouthful!

Because I thoroughly enjoy what I eat I don't go off the rails – except for my one day a month – and my regular evening binges have now stopped completely. This is because I eat a really good meal, and we sit at the table instead of in front of the television. Our evening meal really is quite a social occasion. I can remember the evenings hiding away in the pantry stuffing myself with any food I could lay my hands on because I was still hungry after eating a small dinner! I used to consume thousands of calories between seven and ten o'clock.

Learning that you can eat well but keep your weight steady is a tremendous achievement. One that can make the difference between contentment or misery for the rest of your life.

Dining Out

Eating a large and delicious restaurant meal can often cause a slimmer to worry and wonder whether it is going to be the cause of a possible downfall. I believe dining out is a help not a hindrance to weight maintenance. It does us all good to have food prepared for us – it might be high or low in calories, but because *we* didn't cook it we will never know. If it really is loaded with calories, quite honestly it is better not to know! If I've eaten a large restaurant meal, I rarely eat another meal that day. I select something tempting for a starter, then a substantial dish from the main course (steak rather than fish because then I won't feel hungry later). I will have satisfied my palate with the various gastronomic delights and will feel replete. I might even have a couple of glasses of wine, a small dessert, and a cup of coffee with sugar and cream. Wicked, I know, but not disastrous.

I always avoid two eating appointments in one day because that really would be inviting trouble. Of course I *could* eat the meals and enjoy them, but the next day I would feel hungry at breakfast because often our appetites play games after an overeating session and I'd be putting my self-control under extreme pressure. If such invitations are unavoidable then I would select the menu more thoughtfully, choosing low-calorie items whenever possible. I would drink only one glass of wine and I would skip either the starter or the dessert. Just because I would have to think about what I was eating all the time, I am sure I would not enjoy the meal half as much as if I had only one

31

meal out that day. I must emphasise that I am not suggesting people should have just one meal a day. It is undoubtedly desirable to eat three times a day: breakfast, lunch and dinner. It is a mistake to get too hungry, and you will almost certainly become so if you skip a meal.

One of the biggest downfalls of any weight-conscious person is trying to be *too* good. I have heard of so many slimmers who have nobly selected half a grapefruit as a starter, followed by grilled white fish with green beans as the main course, and finished off with a fresh fruit salad with no cream, only to go home and feel so deprived that they tucked into bread and cheese until they felt really full! There is a psychological desire to feel overfull after you have eaten in a restaurant. If we don't, we feel that we have been shortchanged, and even when we have lost our weight and we are only maintaining our newly found slim figure, we still need the excitement of having overeaten once in a while.

The secret is to select exactly what you fancy from the menu, but to remember that the calorie values of the different dishes vary enormously, and that it does not follow that the more calories that are in a dish the more flavour it will give you. You may enjoy a prawn cocktail just as much as ravioli, but the prawn cocktail will give you a fraction of the calories contained within the fattening, sauce-covered ravioli. We really *don't* have to start the meal with a grapefruit juice. If your passion is a succulent rump steak, then go ahead and order it and enjoy every mouthful, but do realise that just because you have now finished 'dieting' you don't have to go off the rails and choose duck in orange sauce. If you don't mind whether you have a jacket potato or French fries then obviously choose the jacket potato, but if you really adore French fries, go ahead and eat them. When choosing your dessert, try to select something that is fruit-based rather than a cake or pastry dish. Ice cream with hot cherries cooked in brandy has far fewer calories than Black Forest gâteau, for example. Keep reminding yourself that you really *can* eat these things and providing that you cut down a little tomorrow, the extra calories will soon be burnt up.

Many people do not realise which dishes are particularly high or low in calories and therefore do not know what to select for the best. Here are lists of typical starters, main courses and desserts. They have been divided into groups which are low, moderate or high in calorie content so that you can steer a careful course without having to think about individual calories. It is so important to get out of the habit of 'calorie counting', and you can easily learn to automatically 'gauge' particular meals and balance your daily intake accordingly. This is the secret to long-term weight maintenance.

As a general rule, to be on the safe side if you know you are dining out, eat only fruit during that day prior to the meal. This is how my guide to dining out works.

If you select three courses from List A it is doubtful you will gain any weight at all so you can eat moderately during the day of the meal and normally the day after.

If you select two courses from List A and one from List B just make sure you only eat fruit for the other two meals taken that day (e.g. breakfast and lunch or breakfast and supper). Again you shouldn't gain an ounce.

If you only select one course from List A and two from List B, you will need to cut right down before you go out and skip breakfast the following day, eating only fruit that next lunchtime. Twenty-four hours after the extravagant meal you can eat a normal meal.

If you decide to choose something from List C, either the other two courses should be from List A, or better still only have two courses (one from List A) in place of three. If you've only eaten fruit during the earlier part of the day on which you are dining out, there will be little need for remedial action the next day. Skip breakfast by all means, but eat moderately and sensibly for the rest of that day.

Any item on List D is so stuffed with calories that you deserve to starve while your companion enjoys the other courses!

Starters

List A

Select an average portion of one of the following. Do not eat a bread roll, bread and butter or crispbread with your meal.

Artichokes with butter
Asparagus with butter or hollandaise sauce
Bortsch
Chicken noodle soup
Consommé
Florida cocktail
Fresh grapefruit
Fruit juice
Grilled grapefruit with sherry and sugar
Melon cocktail
Mulligatawny soup
Smoked salmon (no bread and butter)

List B

Select an average helping of one of the following. Do not eat a bread roll, bread and butter or crispbread with your meal.

Avocado plus vinaigrette or prawns
Chicken soup with cream
Corn on the cob and butter
Crab mousse
Cream soups
Crudités
Egg mayonnaise
Escargot cooked in butter
French onion soup
Garlic mushrooms in butter
Gazpacho
Ham mousse
Humous
Kipper pâté
Leeks vinaigrette
Melon and Parma ham
Mixed hors d'oeuvres
Mushrooms à la Grecque
Mushroom soup with cream
Oysters
Piperade with croutons
Potted shrimps (no bread and butter)
Prawn cocktail (no bread and butter)
Ratatouille
Ravioli
Rollmops (2)
Savoury choux buns (with cheese)
Shellfish cocktail
Smoked trout
Soup – home-made without cream
Spaghetti bolognese
Stuffed tomatoes (1 large)
Taramasalata (without pitta bread)

List C

Select an average portion of one of the following and only eat bread or toast if it is included on the list. Select other courses from List A if possible.

Any pâté with toast and butter
Moules marinière
Salmon mousse
Smoked mackerel

Taramasalata with pitta bread
Tuna and bean salad
Vol au vents with filling
Whitebait fried

Main Courses

List A

Select an average helping of one item from the list below.

Boeuf en croute
Cauliflower cheese
Cheese omelette
Cheese and potato pie
Chicken chasseur
Chop suey
Dolmades
Filet mignon
Fish – any type grilled or steamed
Fish pie
Fried sweetbreads
Grilled kidneys or with sauce
Ham with mixed salad
Ham omelette with salad
Liver casserole
Mushroom and ham risotto

Pizza, cheese and tomato
Potatoes – jacket potatoes filled with salmon, cream and chives, cottage cheese, pickle or bacon
Shepherd's pie
Sole Véronique (with cream and grapes)
Spanish omelette
Steak tartare (7oz/175g)
Stuffed marrow
Stuffed peppers
Sukiyaki
Tandoori chicken
Tripe and onions
Wiener schnitzel

ACCOMPANIMENTS TO LIST A

Average portions of any vegetables, boiled or raw and served without butter or cream dressings, may accompany any of the above unless the accompaniments are stated. Boiled rice is allowed in place of potatoes where desired.

List B
Select an average helping from the list below.

Beef curry
Bouillabaisse
Cheese and onion pie
Chicken casserole
Chicken pie
Chicken pilaf
Chicken risotto
Chicken – roast
Chilli con carne
Cornish pasty
Croque monsieur
Glazed baked gammon
Indonesian beef satoy
Kebabs – any kind
Lamb chops (2 small grilled)
Lancashire hotpot
Leeks and ham au gratin

Lobster thermidor
Macaroni cheese
Moussaka
Pork chops (1 large)
Potato – baked, stuffed with cheese
Quiche lorraine
Ravioli
Roast beef and Yorkshire pudding
Salmon and hollandaise sauce
Spaghetti bolognese
Steak – grilled (8oz/200g) with salad
Sweet and sour prawns in batter
Toad in the hole

ACCOMPANIMENTS TO LIST B

Average portions of any vegetable may accompany the above dishes. No butter should be added to cooked vegetables. Salads may accompany any dish where desired in place of cooked vegetables, but eat only small quantities of cream–salad accompaniments, e.g., Waldorf salad, potato salad, Russian salad, coleslaw, etc. See recipes for lower-calorie alternatives. If possible select boiled potatoes or boiled rice, but French fried potatoes may be eaten in moderation. Avoid fried rice.

List C
Select one average helping from the list below.

Beef goulash
Beef stroganoff
Boeuf bourguignon
Boiled beef and dumplings
Carbonnade of beef
Cassoulet

Cheese soufflé
Chicken kiev
Chicken paprika
Chow mein
Coq au vin
Crown roast lamb

Duckling à l'orange
Fish and chips
Fried scampi and tartare
   sauce
Lamb biriani
Lamb kebabs
Paella
Peppered steak and cream
   sauce
Pork in cider

Pork pie and salad
Pork – roast
Ploughman's lunch
Prawn biriani and chutney
Steak with French fried
   potatoes
Steak and kidney pie
Sweet and sour pork
Trout with almonds
Veal and ham pie

ACCOMPANIMENTS TO LIST C

Select appropriate accompaniments, but consider the consequences! If you can economise on these, please do so.

List D

Must you select from this list? If so you're obviously determined to be very naughty! Perhaps you should cancel the dinner date! Seriously, think again before going ahead. You know how miserable you'll feel and there are *lots* of alternatives to choose from. You've done so well – don't spoil it now.

Cheese fondue
Chicken with almonds
Chicken koorma

Chicken Maryland (with
   banana, corn fritter and
   bacon)
Game pie
Lasagne

Desserts

List A

Select an average portion of one of the following.

Apples – baked in sugar and stuffed with dried fruits etc.,
   served with a little cream
Fresh fruit salad (6oz/150g) no cream
Ice cream (3oz/75g) any flavour
Loganberries (8oz/200g) with a little cream
Raspberries (8oz/200g) with a little cream
Sorbet (average portion) – any flavour
Strawberries (8oz/200g) with a little cream

List B
Select an average portion of one of the following.

Apple pie (6oz/150g plain or
    4oz/100g with cream)
Banana and custard
Banana split with a little
    cream
Blancmange with no cream
Caramel oranges with no
    cream
Cherries with ice cream and
    brandy
Chocolate mousse
Chocolate soufflé
Chocolate profiteroles
Crème caramel
Fruit fool
Lemon meringue pie

Meringue nest filled with
    fresh fruit and cream
Oranges in cointreau
Peach Melba with a little
    cream
Pears in red wine
Queen of puddings
Rice pudding
Sherry trifle
Strawberries with sugar and
    cream
Summer pudding
Treacle tart – no cream or
    custard or 4oz/100g with a
    little cream
Zabaglione

NB:

If any of the above are eaten with additional cream they
should be treated as an item from List C.

List C
Select one item, but as small a portion as possible. Try to
avoid items on this list.

Apple pie with cream, ice
    cream or custard
Baked Alaska
Bakewell tart
Banana flambée
Black forest gâteau
Bread and butter pudding
Charlotte russe
Cheesecake
Cheese and biscuits
Christmas pudding
Crème brûlée
Crêpes suzette
Danish pastries

Fruit crumble
Rum baba
Sponge pudding (any kind)
Strawberry shortcake
Syllabub
Treacle tart with cream or
    custard

Everyday Meals

For everyday meals, to maintain your weight choose from the following sample menus, bearing in mind what you are planning to eat for your other meals during the day.

Breakfasts

Being Good

Unlimited tea or coffee (no sugar)
½ grapefruit plus any one of the following:
1½oz/40g grilled bacon plus 3 grilled tomatoes
1 Weetabix plus milk and sugar
1 carton natural yoghurt plus 1 teaspoon honey
Small tin of tomatoes on toast
1 boiled egg plus 1 slice toast with low-fat spread
1 slice of toast spread with low-fat spread plus 1 teaspoon
    marmalade or honey

Being Moderate

Small glass unsweetened fruit juice
Porridge (made with water) with milk and 1 teaspoon sugar
    plus any one of the following:
2oz/50g bacon plus tomatoes (unlimited)
1oz/25g bacon and fried egg
Small tin tomatoes, 1oz/25g bacon plus small tin baked beans
1 boiled egg with 4 Ryvitas plus low-fat spread or 1 slice toast
    plus 1 teaspoon marmalade
1 egg scrambled or poached plus 1 slice toast
2 tablespoons muesli plus milk
1½oz/40g any cereal plus milk and sugar

Breakfasts to Be Avoided

Sausage, egg, bacon and tomato plus mushrooms
Kidneys, tomatoes, fried bread
Grilled kippers, bread and butter
Croissant, butter, jam

Snack Lunches

Being Good

Cup of soup (low calorie) and 1 carton natural yoghurt, plus 3 pieces fresh fruit (any kind)

2 thin slices from large wholemeal loaf spread thinly with low-fat spread and made into a sandwich with lettuce, cucumber, tomato, slice of Spanish onion, 1oz/25g ham plus either 1 teaspoon pickle or low-calorie salad dressing (e.g., Waistline)

Large salad with 1 egg and 1oz/25g Edam or lower-calorie cheese (e.g. Shape or Tendale). 1 tablespoon low-calorie salad dressing

Small tin baked beans on 1oz/25g slice toast, low-fat spread

1oz/25g cheese toasted on 1oz/25g slice toast plus two tomatoes

1 egg poached or scrambled on 1oz/25g slice toast plus 1oz/25g tomato

4 Ryvitas, low-fat spread plus 1oz/25g cheese and pickle and tomatoes

4oz/100g ham, tomatoes plus green salad. 1 tablespoon low-calorie salad dressing

5oz/125g chicken joint with tomatoes plus green salad

Low-calorie soup plus fruit yoghurt plus 1 piece fruit

1 small packet crisps plus two pieces fresh fruit

6oz/150g prawns plus salad plus low-calorie salad dressing

4oz/100g carton cottage cheese (with added low-calorie ingredients, if desired) plus large salad or 4 Ryvitas or similar crispbread

Moderate Lunches

1. 3 slices bread (3oz/75g) made into sandwiches with two of the following fillings plus green salad if desired:
     1 egg plus tomato
     1oz/25g cheese plus tomato and pickle
     2oz/50g ham
     2oz/50g chicken or turkey
   2oz/50g salmon plus cucumber
   3oz/75g prawns plus salad
   1oz/25g roast pork plus one item of any fresh fruit (4oz/100g approx).

2. Fried egg plus 4oz/100g chips plus 1 piece fruit.

3. 2-egg omelette filled with tomatoes or mushrooms plus 2oz/50g chips plus 1 piece fruit.

4. 1-egg omelette with 1oz/25g cheese plus salad plus 1 piece fruit.

5. 6oz/150g beans on 1 slice toast plus 2oz/50g ice cream plus 1 piece fruit.

6. Soup plus 1oz/25g bread, egg salad plus 1 piece fruit.

7. Large salad including lettuce, tomatoes, carrots, cucumber, coleslaw, egg, 6oz/150g chicken joint (4oz/100g flesh only), or 4oz/100g ham, with low-calorie dressing plus two pieces fruit or 8oz/200g strawberries plus 1oz/25g single cream.

8. 1 grated eating apple, 1oz/25g sultanas, ¼oz/7g flaked almonds, 1oz/25g chopped dried apricots, ½oz/15g dry oats, ½oz/15g natural bran flakes, mixed with carton natural yoghurt.

9. Ploughman's lunch with 1oz/25g cheese and no butter.

Alternative lunches could be chosen from the list of the moderate breakfasts, and you can add a piece of fresh fruit too. If you are eating lunch in a restaurant you should be able to find the dish of your choice within the guide to eating out. If you are to eat again in the evening, try to select your menu from List A and only eat two courses.

Entertaining at Home

If you are being entertained at a friend's house you must obviously eat what is offered, but of course you don't need to go back for second helpings no matter how delicious a particular speciality may have tasted. Have a good average helping for each course and thoroughly enjoy it. Having learned from the above lists of menus you will know into which category the particular recipes fall. On the other hand, if you are creating your own menu for guests at home you can easily decide on dishes which you know are not too heavy on the calories.

I love entertaining at home, but one rule that I learnt many years ago was not to have three hot courses which required constant nursing to ensure that they did not pass their prime. A hostess should be available to entertain her guests in between adding the final touches to the one course that needs later attention. To be able to prepare a cold starter well in advance of the dinner party leaves you free to concentrate on the main course. Ideally, the sweet can be prepared in advance too, and only the final touches added before serving. There is no need for your guests to have the slightest clue that your menu has been carefully calorie controlled.

Some of my favourite recipes for starters and sweets are given in the recipe section (pages 120–35). If you economise on these two courses then you can prepare anything you like for the main course. Also remember that double cream is exactly what it says – double the calories of single cream. I never use double cream in my cooking, and if I have to use thick cream I would use whipping cream. For sauces I find single cream works perfectly. Always grill rather than fry, or spit roast if you have the facility. Never add butter or margarine to your creamed potatoes, just use ordinary milk. Skimmed milk should be used in place of whole milk in cooking, and meat trimmed of fat before cooking and fat drained from its juices before making any sauces. Eat as many vegetables as you can, but there is no need to lace them with butter.

Drinking While Entertaining

It took a little while to discover that the more I drank the weaker my willpower became, so I now adopt the ruling that I start my evening on simple slimline mixers. I drink wine with my meal and maybe finish with a liqueur. Not only do I stay sober for longer, but my self-control usually

lasts the meal. If you are trying to be particularly economical with the calories a tip which works beautifully for
me is to only have half a glass of wine at a time. This way
your glass is topped up at the same time as everyone else,
but you are only drinking half the quantity. This avoids
your having to say 'no thank you' when your glass is
empty and everybody else is having refills.

Holidays

When many people go on holiday they often feel they must
eat every penny's worth of food that was included in the
holiday brochure price! Often little thought is given to the
result of a whole week of gorging; for instance, eating
three-course breakfasts when normally half a slice of toast
is gobbled down as we run for the bus!

The rules for eating when on holiday are similar to
those when eating out. Remember that if you enjoy a large
meal in a restaurant at night you will normally cut down
the next day. It therefore follows that if you continually
eat out every night for a week or two, you will obviously
gain weight unless you take remedial action at other times
of the day.

By all means eat a cooked breakfast and enjoy the
luxury of it being prepared for you, but select grilled
bacon and tomatoes and maybe a fried egg, skipping the
cornflakes, toast and marmalade. If you have a glass of
orange juice then you really don't need three cups of coffee
too. One of the benefits of being away on holiday is that
you are not continually in the kitchen preparing meals at
all kinds of unusual times for the various members of your
family. Many of my slimmers have come back from
holiday having eaten three square meals a day but have,
in fact, lost weight! Presumably they nibble continually
during a usual day at home. However, *you* are the only
person that knows how you *normally* behave in the pantry
or at work, and you must therefore bear this in mind
whilst on holiday. If you are going on long walks or rock

climbing then obviously you will burn up more calories than sitting behind your office desk. On the other hand, remember that a ten-mile walk in the fresh air works wonders for the appetite!

Many people could learn the best lesson of sensible eating by following the habits of their partners when away from home. Often it isn't your husband who says 'Shall we go in here and have a cup of tea and a cream cake?' Obviously the children think it's a great idea and become very enthusiastic when mum makes the suggestion. The slim husband patiently sits as everyone tucks in and he sips at his cup of tea, probably with no sugar, until everyone has finished. Upon returning home from holiday we wonder why we have gained weight and the others have not. The answer is obvious. The children can accommodate the extra food because they are growing and they are far more active than an adult will ever be. So just think twice before suggesting that you pop into the 'Singing Kettle'!

4
Feeling fit

One of the most wonderful feelings in the world is getting up in the morning, filled with excitement at the prospect of the day ahead. There may be nothing special to look forward to, but you actually *feel* good. If you are feeling fit, relaxed and happy in your mind, and content with your body, you can bounce around doing the housework, enjoy the company of your children and smile as your dog chases a butterfly in the garden. You make your milkman happy by giving him a lovely smile, and you honestly feel on top of the world. Many people will never experience such contentment, but then many people are too concerned about unnecessary trivia to stop and realise how good it is to feel fit.

I apologise if this all sounds rather patronising, but having suffered with asthma since I was a baby I appreciate, possibly more than many, how good it is to feel well. Despite the fact that I still need the aid of inhalers and tablets to curb my breathlessness, twice a week I teach Slimobility exercises to a hundred or so ladies. I would never have believed that I could have built up my level of fitness to such a degree that I am probably fitter than most of my completely healthy members. By designing my own method of dance/exercise movements to tone the body as well as get fit, I have achieved a level of fitness I never believed possible and I enjoy every moment. It is therefore possible for almost everyone to increase their level of fitness and enjoy a healthier life. Even those who are restricted to a wheelchair or have only a minimal amount of movement can still find ways of increasing their fitness level, but it takes regular practice.

So many potential get-fitters who are completely able-bodied make the mistake of believing that unless their fitness campaign is painful, boring, inconvenient or very expensive it isn't going to work. They also believe that they must achieve Olympic standards within a week! When they don't, and they strain a ligament or pull a muscle, they blame the injury for their failure. Achieving fitness is rather like achieving slimness: it takes time and patience. It doesn't need to be too technical which often causes it to become boring; nor does it need to be difficult or too ambitious. If it is you may become disillusioned or could very easily injure yourself. I have met a lot of people outside my classes who have over-energetically attempted to get fit, but have ached so much for the following two days or even a week that they have abandoned the whole project on the basis that 'it's not for me'. So it is vital if you are going to get fit that you attempt it the right way.

When I started taking exercise classes in 1977 I was very unfit, but it was only a matter of weeks before I built up my stamina and strength significantly. I had always been quite supple from dancing as a child and learning yoga as an adult, but until then I could certainly not be considered at all fit. The exercise routines we performed in class were enjoyable, moderately energetic and everyone's body shape improved including my own. However, it eventually seemed as though we were not progressing any further forward or getting a great deal fitter. In 1982 I appointed a new class tutor in Leicester. He was our first male lecturer and his previous training had been as a football trainer, physiotherapist and masseur. After watching him work at his class I realised that there was enormous scope for increasing the level of stamina, strength and suppleness in a way which was great fun. I steered a path between my original methods and those taught by Ted, our male lecturer. These weren't keep-fit exercises, they were get-fit exercises! I called them Slimobility because I designed the movements to specifically tone those areas of the body most likely to suffer from sagging after losing weight. They also dramatically increased the fitness level of our students which enabled them to *feel* better and therefore happier. Because they felt more content they didn't regain their previously lost weight. Also they were able to return to normal eating because they had slimmed on the recommended higher-calorie intake than allowed by most reducing diets. In other words, they had managed to increase or maintain their metabolic rate. They were living proof of my philosophy.

In 1983 it was decided to produce a Slimobility cassette so that students could practise at home as well at the class. I particularly wanted to produce a programme of exercises that fully explained every movement, and was set to 'real' music that could be easily recognised. This was the time when the fitness cassette market exploded and just about every actress or television personality who had a good voice and an enviable figure encouraged you to get fit with them. Jane Fonda was the forerunner and not surprisingly everyone tried to jump on the bandwagon. However, I felt that nearly all of these cassettes and records left a great deal to be desired. There is nothing more frustrating than to stand in your living room adorned with a leotard and feeling a bit silly, to be given lengthy and boring instructions about the cassette, and a detailed explanation of the exercise instruction sheet which usually accompanies them. The verbal instructions were often extremely complicated so that you needed to consult the illustrated instructions, and by the time you had worked out what you were supposed to do the instructor had moved on to the next exercise! How can you get any sense of involvement when you have to break off every two minutes to see what is meant? And anyway, because most people cannot touch their knees with their head or do the splits, it is easy for them to become discontent with their physical state. At the other end of the scale some cassettes contain movements that are so easy and repetitive you don't feel inclined to give them a second hearing. Also, the gaps between the tracks tend to be too long. Therefore, when I was asked to produce Slimobility 1, I was determined to make it so easy to follow that you could just switch it on and know exactly what you were to do next. The music was very carefully chosen to motivate and stimulate the student, and the exercises were very varied with no breaks between the tracks. I felt a sexy male voice would be an added attraction, so I asked Patrick Mower to read the script. What I didn't anticipate was the deep impression he made upon me when I met him for the first time.

I will never forget that day because not only was Patrick even more gorgeous in the flesh than on the television screen, he was extremely charming too. What impressed me most of all was his total professionalism. Despite the fact that he had not seen the script beforehand, he read it with such feeling it sounded as though *he* was performing the exercises personally! The cassette was a great success and we sold many thousands of copies throughout the United Kingdom. Whilst we supplied an illustrated poster with each copy just in case anyone couldn't follow the instructions, it seemed that my plan of totally clear instructions had paid off. We received many letters saying how much students enjoyed using the cassette and I even heard of our competitors buying the cassette and playing it at their own classes! In 1984 we produced a follow-up version – Slimobility 11 – which incorporated more movements and different music. Both cassettes are still available at £4.99 each including postage and packing. If you would like either or both cassettes just send a cheque or postal order made payable to 'SSAGG Mail-Order Account' to the SSAGG Centre, Vaughan Way, Leicester LE1 4SG.

There are a great many different ways of getting fit and in the next few pages you will find exercises to tone up particular parts of your body and to promote stamina and suppleness. Before embarking on any kind of exercise it is wise to check with your doctor if you consider there is any reason why you should not participate in such activity.

For instance, anyone with high blood pressure or a heart complaint could well be advised not to exercise, whereas people with other ailments could benefit from such physical exercise.

Before attempting to exercise, pause for a moment and realise that you have a network of muscles within the body that resemble elastic bands. If you found an elastic band in a cupboard that hadn't been used for many years and you stretched it quite hard it would snap very easily. Realise that if you overwork your body and it has not been worked hard for many years, you could tear a muscle just as easily. Therefore, the importance of warming up completely by undertaking gentle stretching movements is vital, followed by shortened stamina exercises to effect a totally warm body before you become completely involved in your initial routine. Exercise for a short time and do not extend the body too far at the beginning. After you have practised your exercises for some time you should not experience any discomfort, but a feeling of revitalisation. The reason we sometimes ache after not using our bodies for some considerable time is simply because we work our bodies too hard. Various muscle tissues are thought to be involved in this aching sensation, but I would need to devote another chapter to explain the technicalities of this, so no matter how enthusiastic you may feel towards your new fitness campaign, take it gently at the beginning.

Hopefully, after any slightly painful experience from your initial workout, you will find that you do not experience similar discomfort again providing you continue to exercise on a regular basis and at a sensible level. However, to practise gently and regularly for the first week is a far less painful way to start your fitness campaign. You will be delighted at how quickly your body responds as each day goes by and you find that you can perform more exercises with greater ease and with fewer aches the following day.

It must also be realised that our bodies have a natural

alarm system in the form of pain. If at any stage you should feel pain, no matter what kind, you must stop exercising immediately. People often think that if they continue 'the pain will go away'. This is dangerous and stupid and we must learn to listen to our bodies. This particularly applies if we are recovering from an illness or an operation. But on the other hand, it is possible to be too cautious in these circumstances, when in fact practising light exercise could be helpful as an aid to recovery.

The benefits from exercise are not only that you will look better, but it also strengthens the condition of your heart and therefore improves your circulation and can help to prevent coronary heart disease. Research has shown that people who take enough regular exercise can cut their risk of suffering a heart attack, and they may have a better chance of surviving one. Exercise also helps to keep your joints supple as well as your spine, and therefore aids in improving posture. Posture is often one of the first signs of ageing years, and if you can walk well and upright when you are eighty you will look many years younger than your age. When discussing this with my students I often refer to the Queen Mother, who even though she is well into her eighties still walks beautifully upright and looks nowhere near her age. She is a truly remarkable lady.

Exercise also helps to tone up flabby muscles, can give you extra strength, and helps you stay slim. Exercise helps you to cope with stress, and the gently rhythmic exercise found in swimming or cycling is a superb way of releasing tension caused by the strains of everyday life. Your mind and body relax into a rhythm and stress is eased away. Also, the feeling of tiredness, not exhaustion, brought on by physical effort may help promote deep and refreshing sleep.

If you are going to exercise at home it is important to remember the following:
1. Never do strenuous exercises whilst cold – always do an efficient warm-up exercise first.

2. Don't regiment your exercises; use music if possible.
3. Don't invert the body during menstrual periods.
4. Don't take a cold shower after an exercise session; a warm one would be fine.
5. Don't allow yourself to dehydrate during an exercise session; feel free to drink if necessary.
6. Don't push yourself too hard.
7. Give yourself a warm-down session at the end. This can *halve* the time of recovery to normal pulse rate.
8. Relax at the end of your exercises and cool down before replacing your clothes.
9. If by chance you pull a muscle, stop exercising immediately, and as soon as possible place a cold compress on the affected area. Do not apply heat, for example a hot bath, until at least twenty-four hours after the injury occurred. Replace the cold compress every five to six hours if possible, and ensure it is in place for at least fifteen minutes, preferably longer. This will stop any internal bleeding which may be caused by such an injury. If the muscle is pulled in the leg, try to rest it in a raised position so that your toes are level with your nose.

Exercising to Music

It is an interesting fact to realise that exercising to music has the effect of not only making the activity more enjoyable, but it also enables the student to continue practising for longer than they would be able to without the stimulation of a musical accompaniment. It was only recently that I realised personally what a tremendous stimulus music provided. I designed a programme of exercises to be performed daily at home. When I first attempted them they seemed very hard work, but I practised religiously every day. Then one day I bought a new record and played this as I exercised; not only did I not feel so exhausted, but I performed the exercises for twice the number of repetitions. I also enjoyed them much more too, which just goes to prove that often exhaustion is a mental state rather than a physical one!

You may be interested to know the approximate number of calories burned through different sporting activities, divided into aerobic- and anaerobic-type exercises.

The difference between aerobic- and anaerobic-type exercise is simply that in aerobic exercises the energy is generated by oxygen and in anaerobic exercises it is not.

Our muscles are made up of two types of fibres. Slow-twitch fibres (red muscle cells) and fast-twitch fibres (white muscle cells). The red twitch fibres are designed primarily for endurance and stamina work and the white twitch fibres are designed for speed and strength work.

In order to improve your endurance capability you would therefore do the type of exercises that would involve the red twitch fibres in work that would improve their endurance capability. This is done by aerobic- or stamina-type work which is the sort of exercise now being seen to have the greatest advantages in reducing the risk of heart disease and other associated problems, as well as effectively increasing the metabolic rate.

To increase your metabolic rate you need to exercise at an activity level which causes your heart to beat significantly faster. You can calculate your personal *maximum* heartrate by deducting your age from 220. Calculate 60 per cent and 90 per cent of this number, and after a thorough warm-up aim to exercise at an activity level to achieve a heartrate within these levels.

To make sure your heartrate isn't going over the safety limit (90 per cent) and to check that you are working hard enough, you should check your pulse at regular intervals *during* your aerobics class as well as before and after you

---

Facing page: Some of the activities combine aerobic and anaerobic exercises, for example, squash and Slimobility.

Aerobic exercises	Number of calories burned per minute
Badminton – singles	10
– doubles	8
Climbing	12 (approximately)
Cycling	5 to 12 depending on speed
Dancing	3½ to 8 depending on type
Dance – exercise	5 to 7
Football	9
Gymnastics – moving type	6
Jogging	10 (approximately)
Rowing	4 to 11 depending on speed
Running long distance (e.g., marathons)	11
Tennis	7
Skating	7
Skiing – moderate speed	10 to 16
Skiing – uphill, cross country	19
Slimobility exercises	5 to 7
Squash	10
Swimming – breaststroke or backstroke	11 (approximately)
crawl	14 (approximately)

Anaerobic exercises	Number of calories burned per minute
Discus throwing	3
Golf	5
Gymnastics – strength and balancing type	2 to 4
Weightlifting – heavy weights	4
light weights	2
Yoga	2 (approximately)

begin exercising. It is important to take your pulse *immediately* following a maximum activity to find out its effect, as your heartrate falls rapidly as soon as you stop. At this time count your pulse rate over a 10-second period only, and multiply it by 6 thus equalling one minute. When checking your pulse at rest, count over a 15-second period and multiply by 4. For a non-athlete the resting pulse rate would be usually between 60–80 beats per minute. A lower resting pulse rate is generally an indication of fitness, as the heart is pumping the blood around the body more powerfully and efficiently. A top athlete could have a resting pulse rate of around 40 or even lower.

Therefore, in order to improve the fitness factor that will be of most benefit to you, that is your aerobic fitness, aerobic exercises are recommended. Ideally two or three sessions a week of 20–30 minutes should be undertaken. This will ensure a gradual increase in your fitness level.

Anaerobic activity such as weightlifting, the main purpose of which is strength development, can be of some benefit to your general fitness, but by itself it is a poor way to increase your stamina or endurance levels.

So, you should look at the activities that give you the all-round fitness and body toning you desire, and try to find an activity you will enjoy so that you will continue doing it long into the future and gain these benefits for the rest of your life. It would be a mistake to undertake a short-term penance that you are quite likely to abandon after achieving your short-term goal. The benefits of regular exercise are so well established now that it should be an integral part of your everyday life style. Just as this book is designed to help you *stay* slim for ever, physical fitness should be a permanent ambition too.

The S-Factors

True physical fitness is something more than simply being fit to cope with the stresses and strains of everyday life. It consists of three important ingredients – STAMINA, SUPPLENESS and STRENGTH – the S-FACTORS as they are commonly called.

First, and most important is STAMINA. This is staying power, endurance, the ability to keep going without gasping for breath. For stamina, you need a well-developed circulation in the heart and muscles so that plenty of vital oxygen gets to where it's needed. With stamina you have a slower, more powerful heartbeat. You can cope more easily with prolonged or heavy exertion, and you'll be less likely to suffer from heart disease.

Next is SUPPLENESS or flexibility. You need to develop maximum range of movement of your neck, spine and joints to avoid spraining ligaments and pulling muscles and tendons. The more mobile you are, the less likely you'll suffer aches and pains brought on by stiffness.

Finally, STRENGTH. Extra muscle-power in reserve for those often unexpected heavier jobs. Lifting and shifting need strong shoulder, back and thigh muscles. Toned-up tummy muscles also help to take the strain . . . and keep your waistline trim.

The best tests of fitness are those that measure stamina and involve rhythmic movement of large groups of muscles for sustained periods. But people differ in the amount of physical effort they need to make to achieve a reasonable level of fitness. For instance, men must work harder than women; older people should take things more easily.

The Health Education Council's excellent *Looking After Yourself* booklet explains the benefits and also sets out the S-Factor ratings as follows:

The S-Factor scoreboard

	Stamina	Suppleness	Strength
Badminton	★★	★★★	★★
Canoeing	★★★	★★	★★★
Climbing stairs	★★★	★	★★
Cricket	★	★★	★★★
Cycling (hard)	★	★★★	★
Dancing (ballroom)	★	★★★	★
Dancing (disco)	★★★	★★★★	★
Digging (garden)	★★★	★★	★★★★
Football	★★★	★★★	★★★
Golf	★	★★	★
Gymnastics	★★	★★★★	★★★
Hill walking	★★★	★	★★
Housework (moderate)	★	★★	★
Jogging	★★★★	★★	★★
Judo	★★	★★★★	★★
Mowing lawn by hand	★★	★	★★★
Rowing	★★★★	★★	★★★★
Sailing	★★★	★★★	★★
Squash	★★★	★★★	★★
Swimming (hard)	★★★★	★★★★	★★★★
Tennis	★★	★★★	★★
Walking (briskly)	★★	★	★
Weightlifting	★	★	★★★★
Yoga	★	★★★★	★

★	No real effect
★★	Beneficial effect
★★★	Very good effect
★★★★	Excellent effect

Your choice of exercise must also depend on your general state of health. It is stupid to rush into the sort of vigorous exercise that may aggravate a medical condition. And, of course, it depends on how fit you are already.

When you have selected which type of exercise to take, it is important that the correct clothing is worn, particularly footwear. If you are to attend an aerobic exercise class which includes energetic and continuous movements the majority of which are on your feet, light, well-cushioned exercise shoes must be worn to help cushion the jarring of your legs, unless you exercise on mats or a good carpet which will absorb the shock. Wear leg-warmers too, which also help prevent muscle strain as they keep your calves and ankles warm. If you fancy jogging always remember to jog on grass whenever possible, and it is absolutely essential to wear proper jogging shoes. Start off by jogging/walking for 15 minutes, gradually increasing the jogging and decreasing the amount you walk each day. When you can jog continuously for 15 minutes you will be ready to increase your distance.

When undertaking any kind of bending and stretching exercise it is advisable to wear a leotard or catsuit or a loose-fitting jogging outfit or tracksuit. The waistband should never be too tight as this will cause discomfort during your exercises. Loose and comfortably fitting shorts and a sweatshirt or tee-shirt are also ideal for most sporting activities.

The only activity that does not require foot protection is yoga, which should always be practised on your own personal yoga mat. You do not need to go to the expense of purchasing a special one – a piece of plastic foam approximately 6ft × 3ft (2m × 1m) would be ideal, or a piece of carpeting, a folded blanket, or even a sleeping bag, if placed upon a carpet. Choose whatever surface is most comfortable for you, but it should be non-slip.

Pool Exercises

You don't have to be a swimmer to enjoy the benefits of exercising in a swimming pool. Exercising under water adds a completely new dimension to normal exercise as the limbs are worked against the weight of the water and therefore the body works harder. It is also quite hard work keeping your balance, but on the other hand you can enjoy a certain weightlessness. For this reason disabled people often find underwater exercise very useful. Examples of underwater exercises are given below. Except where otherwise stated stand in water to just below shoulder level.

Waist Exercises
1. Hands on hips. Twist 20 times ensuring that your elbows are well below the water.
2. Hands on hips, swivel your hips in an anticlockwise and clockwise direction 10 each way.

Leg and Hip Exercises
1. Hold on to the edge of the pool with your right hand. Swing your left leg, keeping it straight, forward and backward like a ballet dancer. After 10 repetitions with your left leg, turn round and swing your right leg 10 times.
2. Standing in the pool to chest level, raise alternate legs in front of you and touch your foot with your hand. Alternate legs and arms and touch 20 times in total.
3. Holding on to the pool rail facing inwards towards the centre of the pool, draw as big a circle as possible with alternate legs. Practise circling 20 times – 10 each leg.
4. Jog on the spot with water at chest level. 20 steps in total.

5. Jump and allow legs to separate as wide as possible as you land. Arms should go outward too to perform a water jumping-jack. Jump with feet together again and hands down by your side. Perform 10 times.
6. Instead of separating your legs sideways as in 5 perform leg and arm split jumps to the front and back, but do not stop as they come together in the middle. Just jump all the time to allow your legs to go from front to back without a break, and swing your arms forward and backward too. Perform 10 times.
7. Stand as far as possible away from the pool bar, but near enough to hold on to it with your hands. Stretch one straight leg up toward your hands leaving the other stretched well out behind you. Change legs after holding the position for 4 seconds. Repeat 10 times with each leg.

Arm Exercises
1. Stand in the pool so that your shoulders are just submerged in the water. Bend your arms below water level and thrust your elbows back 20 times.
2. Make a paddle with both hands and try to push the water aside as you work them from left to right, 10 times each way. Arms must be straight throughout the exercise.
3. Standing in water at a level just below the shoulders, swing straight arms together in circles. Firstly, make circles backwards 10 times and then reverse the direction and perform 10 times forwards.

Slimobility Exercises

Here are some exercises suitable for an initial warm up to loosen the muscles and increase the amount of blood circulating to them. This minimises the chance of injury. Repeat each position at least 6 times; more if you wish. Practise to music at all times.

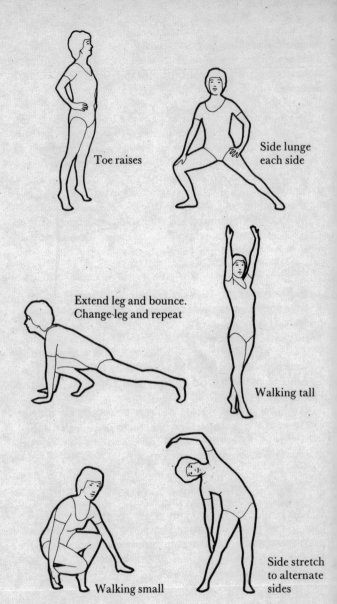

Toe raises

Side lunge each side

Extend leg and bounce. Change leg and repeat

Walking tall

Walking small

Side stretch to alternate sides

60

Aerobic Exercises

These exercises are for a general all over warm-up. Practise to bouncy music and repeat each exercise at least ten times.

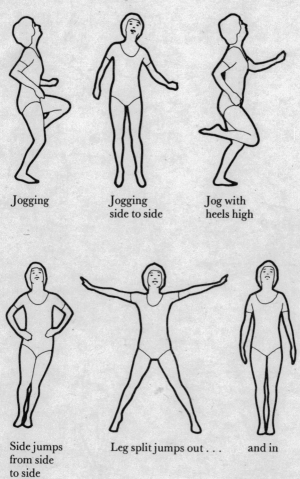

Jogging

Jogging side to side

Jog with heels high

Side jumps from side to side

Leg split jumps out . . .

and in

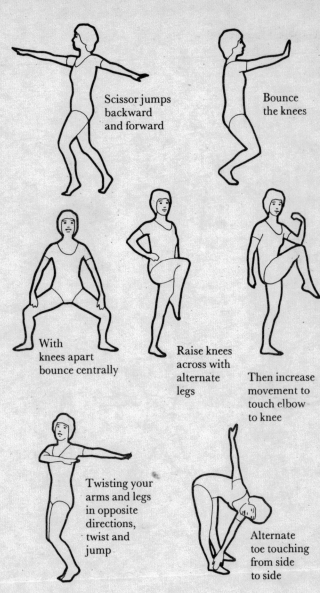

Scissor jumps
backward
and forward

Bounce
the knees

With
knees apart
bounce centrally

Raise knees
across with
alternate
legs

Then increase
movement to
touch elbow
to knee

Twisting your
arms and legs
in opposite
directions,
twist and
jump

Alternate
toe touching
from side
to side

Spot-reducing Exercises

For the Arms, Bust and Shoulders
Practise to any music with a ⁴/₄ tempo. Repeat each
movement at least 10 times.

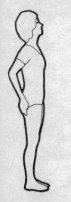
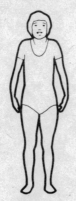
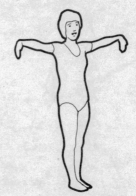

Circle shoulders   and forwards   Arms circling
backwards   with hands down

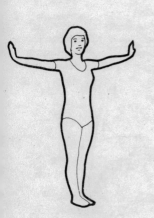
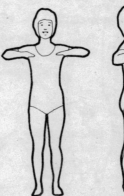

Arms circling   Elbow thrusts
with hands up   forward and back

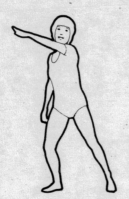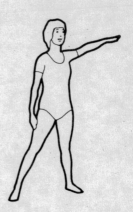

Arm swinging and circling to each side.
Make as wide a circle as possible

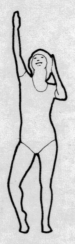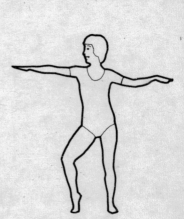

Reach up
really high
10 times

Then stretch
out to sides

For the Waist
Practise as instructed to any music with a ¼ tempo.

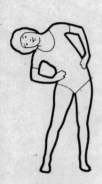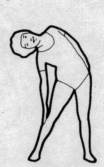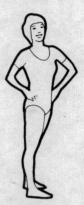

Side bends
twice to
each side.
Repeat 10 times

Side stretch
twice to
each side.
Repeat 10 times

Waist twists
twice to each
side. Repeat
10 times

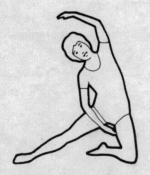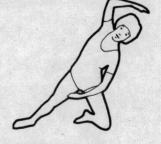

Advanced side bend with leg extended 4 to each side.
Repeat 3 times

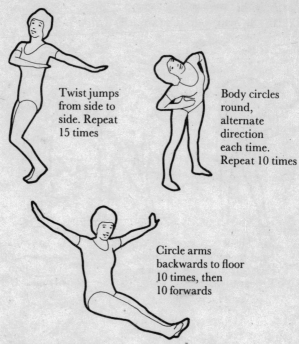

Twist jumps
from side to
side. Repeat
15 times

Body circles
round,
alternate
direction
each time.
Repeat 10 times

Circle arms
backwards to floor
10 times, then
10 forwards

Midriff and Tummy Flattening
Use slower, graceful music. Repeat each action 10 times.

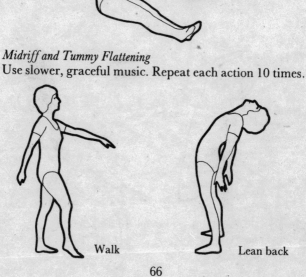

Walk

Lean back

Perform these two exercises together

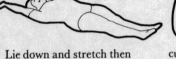

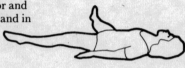

Lie down and stretch then

curl forward so that your head is close to your knees

Raise straightened legs off the floor and swing legs out and in

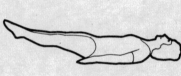

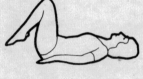

Bend knees in . . .

and out

To Loosen and Strengthen the Spine
Practise to graceful music, preferably with a ¼ tempo.

Bend forward and push hands through your legs

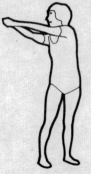

Stand up and swing your outstretched arms sideways

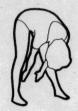

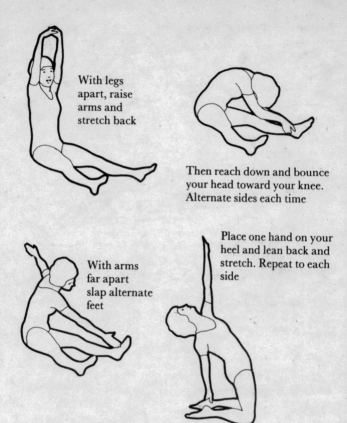

With legs apart, raise arms and stretch back

Then reach down and bounce your head toward your knee. Alternate sides each time

With arms far apart slap alternate feet

Place one hand on your heel and lean back and stretch. Repeat to each side

Arch the spine and curve the spine

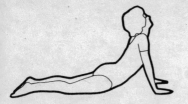 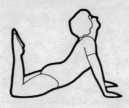

Place weight forward and lower hips. Curl spine and keep head up

Then raise feet behind you

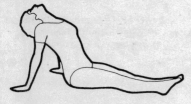 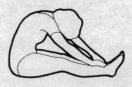

Curve spine upwards

Sit up slowly and relax forward

For Thighs, Hips and Buttocks

Repeat each exercise 10 times and practise to fast-tempo music.

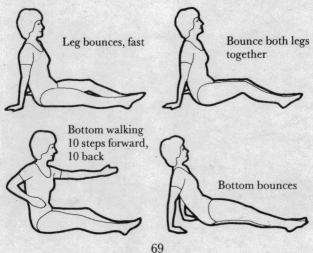

Leg bounces, fast

Bounce both legs together

Bottom walking 10 steps forward, 10 back

Bottom bounces

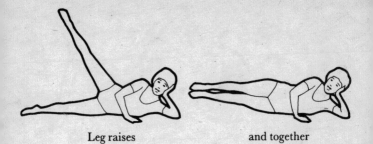

Leg raises   and together

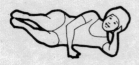

Knee bends and stretch

Roll over after completing these movements on one side and perform the same movements again

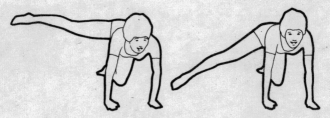

Kneeling on the floor raise leg up . . . and down

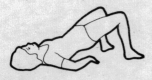

Using your arms and hands to support you, raise your hips and then squeeze knee muscles without altering the position of your legs

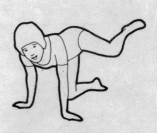

Raise bent leg sideways

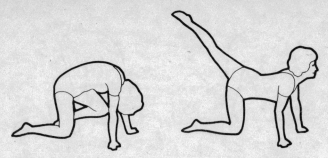

Relax your head down and bring your knee towards your chin, then extend leg and raise head

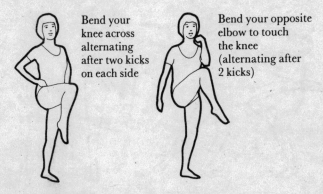

Bend your knee across alternating after two kicks on each side

Bend your opposite elbow to touch the knee (alternating after 2 kicks)

Leg Toning Exercises
Practise to music with a 4/4 tempo and repeat each movement at least 10 times unless otherwise stated.

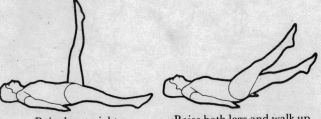

Raise leg straight

Raise both legs and walk up and down

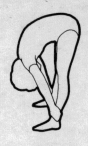

Stretch over to one leg twice then repeat with other leg

Straighten up and stretch down holding both legs

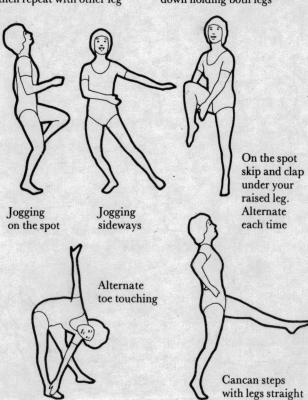

Jogging on the spot

Jogging sideways

On the spot skip and clap under your raised leg. Alternate each time

Alternate toe touching

Cancan steps with legs straight

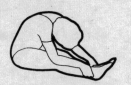

Sit up, stretch forward,
relax head to knees

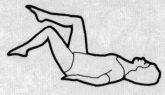

Cycling

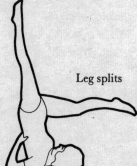

Leg splits

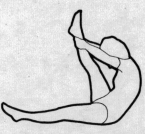

Raise alternate straight legs

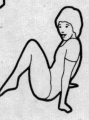

Bend knees, with
toes pointing
to the floor

Keeping the
legs off the floor,
straighten legs

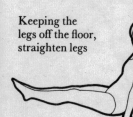

Bounce legs out and in
5 steps each way
and repeat 5 times

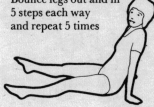

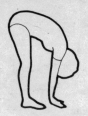
Leg stretch

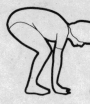
Bounce and straighten

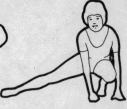
Bounce with leg extended. Change sides

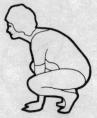
Crouch and bounce

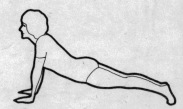
Thrust your legs out and bounce

The Warm Down

It is essential that these exercises are practised after every session, to 4/4 music and without too much energy. Repeat these warm-down exercises as directed.

Gentle side bends. Each side 6 times

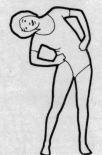

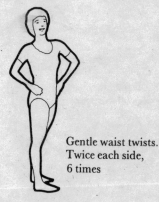

Gentle waist twists. Twice each side, 6 times

74

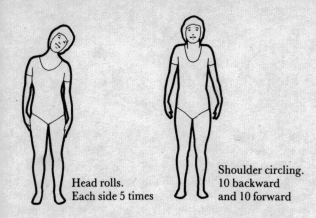

Head rolls.
Each side 5 times

Shoulder circling.
10 backward
and 10 forward

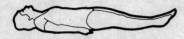

Slowly lie down and relax completely for 5 to 10 minutes

5
Help yourself to love and enjoy sex

If you have been overweight for some considerable time you may have developed a very low self-image of your body. 'How could anyone fancy this great fat lump?' is a familiar thought which no doubt will have crossed your mind when you were feeling particularly despondent about your size. Unfortunately, this low self-image may continue even after achieving a slim figure. Such an inferiority complex can have a far-reaching effect on a personal relationship, and over a number of years this situation can even cause a marriage to break down.

Because the woman *feels* unattractive she may try to avoid the possibility of her husband wishing to make love to her. She may go to bed earlier than usual, complaining that she feels overtired. When her husband retires to bed sometime later she pretends to be asleep. Alternatively, she may complain of having a headache, toothache, tummy ache, or a sore throat. If we don't want to make love we can think of all sorts of excuses to get out of it!

It is an unfortunate fact that sexual habits can decline very rapidly. In other words, the longer you leave between making love, the easier it is to keep putting it off. Some couples go months without sex and think little of it, and even avoid the possibility by rarely kissing and cuddling in bed. I believe that underneath that cool exterior there is a sad and empty feeling of being unloved. It is a vicious circle as the woman who feels unattractive and lacking in self-confidence may appear offhand to her partner which in turn causes him to feel inferior too. He questions his own capabilities, from his standing in the community, to the dimensions and strengths of his sexual assets! This can often result in his looking elsewhere for reassurance. Can you blame him? Of course not. You've probably done nothing to give him confidence or make him feel wanted. It is a natural feeling to want to be loved, and it is a great shame if vanity gets in the way.

It is a common belief that a satisfactory sexual relationship is not particularly important to marriage. In fact, research shows that it is *the* most important single factor. If your physical relationship is successful you are more likely to be closer to your partner mentally too. You are more likely to discuss all manner of subjects, including your figure, and your everyday relationship is likely to be less inhibited. If you are very close you will be a happier person, and the chance of your family being happy is much greater too. But perhaps what is most important to you is the fact that it will help you to slim and stay slim. Making love can certainly help improve your figure by toning up your legs, midriff and hips, and at the end of this chapter I will give examples of exercises that can be practised to help improve your figure and your sex life.

One of the fundamental rules of a satisfactory sexual relationship is the ability to relax. Many people do not relax simply because they feel ashamed of their body. It is essential to forget any bodily imperfections and learn to accept yourself as you really are.

I mentioned in an earlier chapter how it is possible to be considered attractive without an hour-glass figure. Similarly, it is possible to learn the art of becoming sexually attractive without the generally recognised attributes. As I believe very few women would prefer to be unattractive to the opposite sex, let us consider the desires of the majority.

Sexual attraction is difficult to define, but we are led to believe that actresses like Joan Collins, Brigitte Bardot and Victoria Principal have the desired qualities. Strangely, men and women have very differing views of who does and who does not possess sex appeal so it follows that they also differ in their opinion of what is required to achieve it. Women usually believe that super-slim hips and thighs and large breasts are a basic necessity, preferably combined with a perfect hairstyle and a beautiful face. In the hope that they might achieve this perfection they are continually attempting to become unnaturally slim by embarking on crash diets, sleeping in curlers, and plastering their faces with far too much face cream when they go to bed. No wonder sex is dead in many households!

But why do they have to strive for the impossible. Every human body on this planet is unique. We *cannot*, and were not intended to, look like anyone else but ourself. Yes, we can make the most of what we have and this we should do for our own peace of mind, but we must be *sensible* and *realistic*. Learn to relax about your figure – we have all got faults, but it does not mean we are not attractive in our own way. After all, it is the real you your man wants, not an artificial substitute, otherwise he wouldn't have married you or asked you out, so don't pad out your bra with cotton wool, wear a hair piece, or apply your make-up with a palette knife. Let him see the real you, happy and relaxed.

There are, however, lots of things we can do to make us more attractive naturally. Freshly washed hair, not lacquered into a solid mass but allowed to flow easily, for instance. There is nothing that will make you more attractive than a gentle fragrance of perfume, a satin soft skin helped by using body lotion after every shower or bath, and cosmetics carefully applied to accentuate your best facial features. It is important not to overdo your make-up, for although your man will appreciate that you have taken time and trouble to look your best for him it could turn him off if you appear 'untouchable', so make-up should be thoughtfully applied.

If you want to be sexually attractive ensure that your teeth are really clean and that your mouth smells fresh. Any unsightly facial hair should be removed, and all clothing should be freshly laundered. It is essential to use an effective body deodorant and anti-perspirant, but a feminine deodorant is unnecessary; use plenty of soap and water and a little talc instead. If you are a smoker this may very effectively cut down your chances of meeting Mr Right. The Scottish Health Education Council's tee-shirt sums it up perfectly: 'Kiss a non-smoker and taste the difference.'

On the subject of making love, the only advice I would offer is to communicate to each other. Make encouraging noises when you are particularly enjoying one action, but stay quiet if you are not. He will soon learn what you like and together you will soon gain confidence in communicating individual or mutual pleasures. Forget the outside world when making love – that way you can really be yourself – and don't be ashamed of anything you want to do. You and your lover are the only ones to know what suits you. Just enjoy yourselves together – you may be very pleasantly surprised.

If you are already married I hope your sexual relationship with your husband will improve now that you are slim and more self-confident, but remember that he needs your compliments just as much as you need his. Words like 'You're the most wonderful lover' will ring like music in his ears and can only enhance your relationship.

In a new sexual relationship never draw your man's attention to your jodhpur thighs, slightly bulging midriff or stretch marks! I promise he will not notice any of them because he will be far too worried about what you think of *his* body. So stop worrying about yourself and try to learn to relax. Capture his heart by kissing him tenderly and being warm towards him. He will need his confidence boosting too; men like to be told they are attractive, have a beautiful body, lovely hair . . . just as we do.

Listed overleaf are various exercises which can be practised separately which will further increase enjoyment of your sex life.

1. To strengthen and tone up thighs and buttocks lie face downward with your legs together, and raise each leg separately 5 times. Hold for the count of five, then raise both legs together, slowly, and count to five as you hold them as far as possible off the floor. Legs must be absolutely straight at all times.

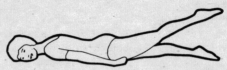

Raise legs individually 5 times each, then together. Hold for 5 seconds

2. Lie on your back and bend your knees, feet a little way away from your body. Raise your hips off the floor and squeeze your legs together. Repeat 20 times.

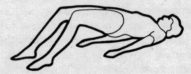

Raise hips off floor and squeeze legs together

3. Maintain the same position as 2 above, but tense and relax your hips and buttock muscles. Repeat 20 times.

4. Lying on the floor facing upward with your legs outstretched in front of you, tense and relax your vaginal muscles. This can be achieved by contracting the muscles that control the actual opening. Relax, then repeat the contraction again. Repeat the contractions 20 times.

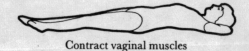

Contract vaginal muscles

5. Lie on your tummy and place your hands straight out in front of you. Raise your arms and legs a short distance without straining. Keep your legs as straight as possible. Hold the position initially for 2 seconds. As your back and abdominal muscles strengthen increase the time you hold your body so that ultimately you can hold the pose for 10 seconds without any strain. Perform once only.

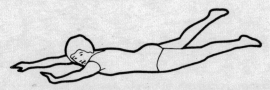

Raise your arms and legs and hold for 2 to 10 seconds

6. Lie on your back and bend your legs so that your feet are approximately 2ft (·75m) away from your body. Raise your hips as high as possible and then lower them back to the floor. Initially raise your hips only five times, holding for the count of three, increasing the repetitions as you get stronger to 15 times, holding for 5 seconds.

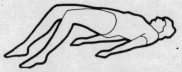

Raise and lower hips

7. To strengthen the inner thigh muscles and increase flexibility, sit on the floor with your hands together outstretched behind, your legs as far apart as possible without straining. Stretch your spine and lean over toward one leg, attempting to touch your knee with your head. Hold for 2 seconds. Slowly sit up and relax before performing the exercise to the other side. Prac-

tise twice each side initially, building up to five times. This exercise *must not* be rushed.

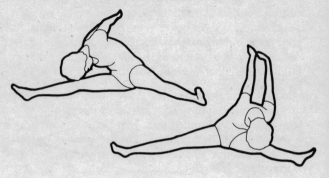

Hands clasped behind your back, stretch head over to alternate legs

6
Looking good

Getting slim after years of struggling with different diets might make you *feel* better, but do you really *look* so much better. A slim but flabby body certainly doesn't, nor does a slim but badly groomed one. Just because your scales tell you that all is well in the weight department does not mean that you don't have to work at other areas so that you actually look terrific.

I have already explained the many benefits of exercise when it is practised regularly, and a fit body, even if it is still a little heavy, can look fantastic. No wobbly bits, but beautifully toned so that it goes in and out in all the right places! This chapter is to help you embark on a total self-improvement campaign. Not only will this act as an insurance policy to protect you against any possibility of regaining weight, but it will help you to achieve your physical potential and complete your new image.

Hair

Perhaps you have kept your same style for years. There is no better way to change your image than to have a new hairstyle.

Everyone is an individual. Face shapes can vary quite considerably due to the arrangement of bone structure, muscle tissue and skin. With the hair being so close to the face it can (and indeed should) be used as one would use make-up – to accentuate the good points and detract from the poor ones.

Before you walk in to your favourite salon with a copy of a magazine illustrating models or movie stars showing off their crowning glory, pause for a moment and ask yourself if your hair is capable of such a style. No hairdresser can easily change naturally curly hair, for instance, into a straight and flowing style. Similarly a thin head of hair would never produce a long, thick curly style. Nature simply didn't intend that style for you. Your hair stylist is experienced and can advise you of the best style to suit your hair and your face shape, but here are some basic guidelines.

The ideal face shape is oval with prominent cheekbones, and a hairstyle should be designed with this in mind.

A round face needs height in the hairstyle, but no width. There should not be a heavy fringe.

A long face needs width and not height. Hair should be no longer than jaw level, and some hair should cover part of the forehead. Do not have a centre parting.

A face with a heavy or square jaw needs lift or width above the eyes. Hair around the jaw will only emphasise the squareness.

As a general rule the higher the parting the longer the face appears. The fuller the fringe, the wider the face appears.

The two most important qualities of lovely hair is condition and the cut. Condition can be improved effectively and quickly by using a conditioner that is suitable for your hair type, for instance, for dry or oily hair. A good, healthy diet is also important. Too much heat or chemical treatments will damage the hair to the point of splitting or breaking. Split ends can only be cured by being cut off. If you become unwell at any time this will have a detrimental effect on the behaviour of your hair, too. Although it is necessary to have professional treatment for cutting and other technical services, most women can deal with their hair at home between visits to the hairdresser. Depending on the way the hair is handled, much unnecessary damage can be caused so think about prevention rather than cure.

Take note of the following points:

Do not use excessive heat – curling tongs or hot brushes or heated rollers should not be used too often. Do not hold your hair dryer too close, or expose hair to strong sunlight or even ultraviolet light.

Do not use damaging tools – metal combs, rough-edged plastic combs or extra-hard nylon brushes.

Do not sleep in rollers.

Do not grip or pin the hair constantly in the same place – rubber bands are particularly damaging.

Do not pull hair tangles when the hair is wet.

Do use conditioners to lubricate the ends.

Do use good-quality combs and brushes.

Do cover the hair when you are in extreme weather conditions (e.g., strong sunlight, blustery winds).

Remember that shampooing plays a large part in the conditioning process.

The following ideas can combine to make the correct formula for the individual:

Oily hair (and scalp) needs washing every 2 to 4 days. Use a liquid shampoo, one application only. It is a good idea to dilute the shampoo first. Always use tepid, not hot, water and do not massage the scalp. Instead rub lightly with the flat of the hand.

Dry hair (and scalp) needs washing every 6 to 8 days. Use a cream shampoo, one application only. Try to create a lather before applying and use warm water to stimulate the scalp. Massage the scalp thoroughly with your finger tips and rinse carefully. Use conditioning creams whenever possible.

Normal hair (and scalp) needs washing every 4 to 6 days. Use variation between dry and oily treatment.

Combination hair that is oily at the roots and dry at the ends (usually long hair) is generally better if treated as dry hair, otherwise the ends become overwashed and 'fly away'. After a while it may be necessary to change the 'formula', or products used, as the scalp can become immune to the action of just one.

Colouring and permanent-wave products are now more readily available for home use. If these are going to be used it should be remembered that they are chemicals, some quite harmful, and should be treated with care. Approximately 80 per cent of heads of hair in poor condition are due to incorrect home-colouring and permanent waving. For colouring, the important rule to remember is that semi-permanent colour will *not* lighten hair at all, and will wash out after about six shampoos. When hair is lightened, even half a shade, this is permanent and the hair will not return to its natural colour except in the new growth. If there are any doubts at all, seek advice from a reputable hairdresser.

It should be borne in mind that if your hairstyle is to change, the following order of events should be followed:

Improve the condition first
Visit your hairdresser for a professional cut or restyle –
    this is *essential*
If your hair is in good condition then colouring could be
    undertaken
If your hair has taken the colour treatment without
    losing any condition, permanent waving could also
    be undertaken

To be an asset, hair must conform to these five points:

It should be the correct shape for the individual
It should be natural looking
It should shine
It should be pleasing to touch
It should have a pleasant smell without being perfumed

Skin Care

Basic Principles of Skin Care
Everyone, no matter what their skin type, should cleanse, tone and moisturise their skin every single day.

If you wear no more make-up than lipstick you should still cleanse, tone and moisturise. If you cleanse your face at night then a skin food should be applied (that is a night cream), and then a moisturiser applied in the morning. A moisturiser is a protector, not a nourisher.

It is necessary for you to diagnose your skin type.

Symptoms of a dry skin are:

(a) That it sometimes flakes
(b) That it feels taut after washing
(c) That it may be very sensitive
(d) That it may have a tendency to wrinkling

Symptoms of an oily skin are:

(a) A continually shining nose
(b) Open pores (giving the appearance of an orange-peel effect on the skin)
(c) A tendency towards blackheads and spots

You may consider that your skin is what is commonly known as a 'combination skin'. If your skin is dry on the cheeks, but has an oily patch down the centre of the face, i.e., forehead, nose and chin, then your skin falls into this category.

Cleansing
Ordinary everyday soap can be harmful to the delicate skin on your face. Cosmetic soaps are available but are very expensive. Preferably find a cleanser to suit your particular skin type. (Combination skins will have to be treated as two separate skin types.)

Apply cleanser with both hands, gently massaging the face in an upward circular movement. This dissolves any make-up or everyday grime and cleanses the pores. Then remove cleanser completely with damp cotton wool.

Gently remove all eye make-up with an eye make-up remover lotion, but take care not to drag the skin. I find Boots No. 7 eye cleanser ideal, or alternatively I use almond oil on dampened cotton wool.

Toning

This process not only closes pores which have been opened by the cleanser but it also removes any remaining traces of cleansing cream. Many toning products are available, but there is really no need to spend a lot of money when you can make up your own. Always apply with cotton wool.

For a *dry skin* use neat *rose water* (available from Boots at around 90p for 500ml which is enough to last you for about a year).

For an *oily skin* use 2 parts *rose water* and 1 part *witch hazel*. This can be made up for you at the chemist or you can buy a bottle of each and mix your own.

For a *combination skin* use neat *rose water* on *dry* areas and *rose water* and *witch hazel* at a 2:1 ratio (as oily skin) on oily centre panel.

Be very careful not to buy a cheap branded product which may be far too astringent for your skin. A toning lotion should not sting the face; if it does, it is too strong.

Night Creams

After thorough cleansing and toning your face and neck at night, everyone over the age of twenty-eight should apply a small quantity of night cream – one particularly designed for your skin type. Ask the advice of a qualified beautician because you want to be sure you buy the correct night cream as they can be expensive.

Apply cream with the tips of the third fingers (these are the most sensitive) and massage gently into the skin. After 10 minutes the cream will have penetrated into the face and disappeared. Any excess on the skin will be wasted. It pays to be economical with your night cream.

Moisturisers

A moisturiser must be applied every morning whether you follow it with other cosmetics or not. Even if no other cosmetics are worn a moisturiser is essential. It protects the skin from the elements, and also provides a suitable base on to which a foundation cream may be applied, or alternatively, you may prefer to apply just a little powder.

An *oily skin* needs a cream that is light in texture and non-greasy. It will protect the skin from pollution, thus helping to prevent spots.

A *dry skin* needs a fairly oily moisturiser – one that will protect the skin and remain on the surface to provide a smooth base for your make-up. If the wrong cream is used it will disappear into the skin and you will not be able to apply your foundation cream smoothly.

Combination skins should try one moisturiser, applying more to the dry areas. If this is not satisfactory then two separate creams will have to be used.

To sum up:

Cleanse and tone every day.
If over twenty-eight feed the skin nightly with a night cream.
Protect your skin every morning with a moisturiser.

Special Creams
There are many products on the market which are designed for particular problems. These vary from eye creams which can minimise wrinkling and neck creams for the same purpose, to special creams for a dehydrated or tired and generally out-of-condition skin. If you have a particular skin problem it would be money well spent to have a facial by a qualified beauty therapist and to follow her advice. After all we only have one face so we might as well make the most of it!

Face Masks
Depending on your skin type a face mask can help to eliminate spots by thoroughly cleansing the skin. Use according to the instructions described on the particular package. Again, consult your beauty therapist for advice.

Make-up

Each day follow the cleanse, tone and moisturise routine as described under 'Skin Care'.

If you wish to apply make-up, use your cosmetics in the following order:

Moisturiser

Always apply before any make-up as it protects the skin and provides a 'basecoat' or 'undercoat' for your foundation cream, enabling it to be applied smoothly.

Apply your moisturiser all over the face and neck with the finger tips using a gentle movement.

Foundation Cream

Foundation cream adds an even-looking colour to your face and can make a tremendous difference to your appearance. Choose your colour carefully – ask the beauty consultant for advice on shades for your colouring. Apply 'spots' of cream over your face and quickly blend them together with your finger tips, extending the movements up to your hairline, ears and neck. Smooth downwards so that the little hairs which are to be found all over your face will lie in the direction in which they grow. Use an old toothbrush to brush on the edges to your hairline and to brush your eyebrows into place. Remember that foundation creams can be mixed to achieve the ideal shade.

Lipstick

Apply lipstick carefully, preferably with a lip brush (available from chemists or a beauty counter in a large store). If you wish, you may add lip gloss afterwards.

Blusher

Blusher adds a delightful glow and enhances the shape of your face. Available in powder form or as a cream, apply blusher just below cheekbones and blend in carefully. If you wish to use face powder, apply cream blusher before the face powder or powdered blusher afterwards. Seek advice from a beautician on suitable shades.

Powder (optional)

Powder helps to set your make-up so that it lasts longer and also helps to provide a matt finish, often desirable for ladies with an oily skin. Apply loose powder with a clean piece of cotton wool. Dab it all over the face pressing rather than rubbing. Brush off excess with cotton wool or a large clean cosmetic brush. Try a translucent shade which is colourless but allows the colour of your foundation to show through.

Eye Shadow

The purpose of eye shadow is to make your eyes appear larger, as well as making them prettier.

Various colours of eye shadow can be combined to create a pretty but subtle effect. For a total eye make-up apply a base of very light shadow (beige or cream) all over the eye area – i.e., from below the eyebrow to above the eyelashes. Then apply a light-coloured eye shadow on the inner corner of the eyelid, and then upwards and outwards with a darker shade. Blend it in carefully. Eye shadows are available in many different forms. Experiment to find which type you prefer: powder, cream or liquid shadow. Boots sell an effective eye foundation cream which prevents creasing and is inexpensive.

Eyeliner

This is one cosmetic that is often left out but helps to make your eyes look larger and your lashes longer and thicker. Apply a thin line next to the upper lashes, from the inner corners to the outer corners. If you wish, you may also apply a very thin line below the lower lashes, but only from the centre outwards (not the full width). There are several excellent eyeliners available which include a very fine brush to ensure easy application.

Alternatively, use one of the new extra-soft eye pencils which can be applied very close to the eyelashes or even inside the lashes.

Mascara

Apply mascara to upper and lower lashes as desired. A spiral brush ensures easy application separating the lashes while coating them with mascara. This makes them look thicker and longer. Try applying your mascara using zig-zag movements with the brush. This helps separate the lashes and avoids clogging. If you are not used to making-up, spend lots of time practising.

Only by experimenting will you be able to find the most attractive 'design' for your face.

Make-up should create a beautiful illusion, so try not to overdo it. If you wear spectacles, remove them while applying face make-up and lodge them on the end of your nose while you apply your eye make-up.

After completing your make-up you should feel and look much better.

Underwear

Well-fitting underwear can make a tremendous difference to your figure, so it is worth taking a little trouble to find the correct size and style for your particular shape.

A bust need not be flat to warrant a slight padding to give a good shape and uplift and put fullness where it is most needed. Heavier bustlines and ladies with midriff bulges will find a long-line bra a great help. Very few women wear the correct size bra – they measure themselves round the fullest part of the bustline and take potluck as to cup size. Very much a trial and error situation.

The correct way to measure yourself is underneath the bust (around your back and ribcage). Add 5 inches to that measurement and you will have your bra size. For example, if you measure 31 inches with the tape measure, add 5 inches to make 36 inches. You would need a 36-inch bra. Now measure yourself around the fullest part of your bust. If that measurement is the same as the first measurement (including the 5 inches) you need a small or A cup; 1 inch larger indicates a medium or B cup; 2 inches more indicates a large or C cup; 3 inches indicates an extra full or D cup.

Always try on a bra before buying it unless you purchase it from a store which will readily exchange the garment or refund your money. The Playtex Cross-Your-Heart bra or a similar-style bra by Marks & Spencer works wonders for the figure, even though they may not be particularly pretty.

Pantie girdles can flatten your tummy, but often create huge bulging thighs! You may well look better not wearing one at all. If they are worn continually you may find that thick thighs develop and your waistline disappears. Similarly, bikini panties if worn too tight, can create bulges on the hips which will remain after the panties have been removed. Better to buy a size larger so that they don't cut into the flesh.

Some older ladies find an all-in-one foundation garment a great help. You may be lucky enough to find a make which really fits you properly with the bra positioned in the right place. Otherwise you will have to have one made to measure. They are expensive but do a first-class job. Alternatively, buy a long-line bra and combine it with a high-line girdle.

To sum up:

Make sure you are wearing the correct bra size for your figure

Only wear a girdle if you really feel it does something for you – avoid them if possible

Don't wear panties that are too tight

If you wish to wear a one-piece foundation garment, make sure it fits *everywhere*.

Dress Sense

Having lost all or at least the majority of your weight you will be determined to look good in the clothes you wear. However, many ladies, whether overweight or slim, select the wrong style, when they could easily camouflage any figure faults by clever dressing. A problem which often affects the lady who has just become slim after many years of being overweight is that she cannot get used to being slim. She still goes to the size 16 or 18 dresses instead of her proper size of 10 or 12. It is a habit many find difficult to drop.

Here are some golden rules which I hope you will find helpful.

1. Always aim to achieve a 'total' look. If your outfit is up-to-the-minute fashionwise then your accessories should be too.
2. Accessories should always match, i.e., black shoes, black handbag and black gloves (though if you wish you could wear gloves which are the same colour as your outfit).
3. Shoes should either match your outfit or be darker. White shoes can be very unflattering to the feet unless they are strappy sandals worn with a white summer dress or trousers.
4. Your coat or dress should be the main attraction, with your accessories complementing it. The exception to this rule is, of course, a special hat worn for a wedding. When buying a hat, ask the sales lady to demonstrate how it should be worn.
5. When shopping for accessories take your outfit with you to compare the colour, suitability, style etc., and if in doubt, don't buy!
6. When choosing something to be worn during the day, judge it in daylight. If it is to be worn in the evening, then make sure that you see yourself in artificial lighting before you decide to buy.

7. Stand back from the mirror and assess the co-ordination of the colours of an outfit at a distance. It is the *general* look which is important.
8. After a special occasion has taken place, don't put your new outfit away never to be worn again until another special occasion. It is too good to waste and as time passes it will become out of date and your figure may change. *Wear* it while it looks at its best and enjoy looking good.
9. When choosing clothes it helps if you can diagnose your figure type.

   There are three categories:

   Hippy
   Busty
   Roly-poly

   (a) Hippy figures look much better in A-line skirts with any patterns or details worn above the waist, not below it. Try to wear darker colours below the waist and lighter colours or patterns above it.

   (b) The reverse applies to busty figures. Often people with heavy busts have delightfully slim hips and legs and look splendid in pleated skirts and in trousers, but they should wear plain dark colours above the waist if they wish to minimise their bust size. Avoid low necklines.

   (c) Roly-poly figures should be dressed in plain fabrics and styles should always be simple too. No belts, frills or pleats as these only have the effect of making the figure look rounder!
10. Generally speaking dark colours are more slimming, pastel shades are more flattering to the more mature woman, and if you want to be noticed, wear red. Black and white accentuate your face so your make-up and hair must be perfect, and avoid these colours if you are feeling under the weather.

    Wear white- or natural-coloured underwear under white blouses, sweaters, etc. Wear black or natural coloured underwear under black garments, particularly if they are see-through.

11. If you feel the cold try to buy dresses with long sleeves rather than wearing a cardigan to keep you warm. A long-sleeved dress is much smarter.

12. Woolly hats are much smarter than headscarves.

13. Whatever you are wearing should always look like an outfit. Don't mix patterns unless they match; always wear a plain blouse with a patterned skirt, and so on. Try not to mix textures either. Wear wool with wool and cotton with cotton.

14. Plan your wardrobe in advance so that you can make the most of what you buy. It may be a good idea to buy one accessory each time you buy a major item. This way you soon build up a wardrobe of accessories enabling you to look really smart all the time.

Nail Care

To appear well groomed not only does your hair need to look clean and tidy, your make-up add something to your beauty, and your clothes help to give the illusion of a perfect figure, but your nails need to look well cared for too.

Nails do not need to be painted to look good. So long as they are the right length and are really clean, they will look fine.

If you want to give yourself a proper manicure your kit should include:

Nail polish remover (if necessary)
A small bowl of warm soapy water and a small towel
An emery board
Cotton wool
Orange stick
Cuticle cream/remover
Hand cream
Base coat (optional)

Nail enamel (optional)
Nail enamel setting oil or an aerosol spray-dry product
(optional)

Manicure Routine
Assemble everything on a tray
Remove enamel with remover
File nails with an emery board, never a steel file. File in
one direction only: towards the centre tip of the nail
Shape the nail into an almond shape
Wash hands – this removes filings and makes cuticles
softer
Dry well
If the cuticles need special attention brush cuticle oil/
remover round the cuticles and press back with an
orange stick (hoof end) covered with a tiny bit of cotton
wool. Remove dry skin from nail only. Never cut your
cuticle as it protects the unborn nail which starts at
your first knuckle. If the cuticle is cut, germs can creep
into this delicate area and cause infection.
Wash hands again and brush nails. Dry carefully.
Apply plenty of hand cream.
Wipe nails with cotton wool or a tissue to remove all traces
of any grease from the hand cream.
Use nail strengthener at this stage if your nails are brittle.
Ask your chemist for advice.
Apply a base coat varnish. This acts as a primer and evens
the surface of the nail. It helps the varnish to stay on
better, and it provides a colourless barrier between your
nail and a dark-coloured varnish, thus preventing
possible discolouration by a very strong-coloured
enamel.
Apply nail varnish. Be adventurous with colours. There
are hundreds to choose from.
Coat brush with just enough varnish so that it doesn't
flood off the end. Re-dip for every nail. If you are
right-handed, apply to right hand first, starting at the
little finger and working towards the thumb. If you are

left-handed – vice-versa. Apply three strokes to each nail. Centre first, then either side. After painting each nail remove a hairline edge from the nail tip by wiping it along the side of your thumb; this helps to prevent varnish lifting and cracking. Apply two coats of plain varnish or three of frosted or pearlised. Always allow to dry for about 5 minutes between coats so as to avoid smudging. When the last coat is almost dry, apply enamel dryer and then sit back and relax for 5 minutes.

It takes 12 hours for your varnish to set really hard. The best time to manicure your nails is last thing at night. Worst enemies to newly painted nails are sharp objects and hot water. Try to avoid these whenever possible.

Tips for Hands and Nails

Wear rubber gloves when doing the washing or washing-up.

Wear old leather gloves for gardening jobs.

Use hand cream after hands have been in water. Carry hand cream in a small container in your handbag. Keep some by the sink and at your place of work. Use as much as your hands will absorb.

Use a thimble when sewing.

Always dry your hands thoroughly – dampness encourages chapping.

Give yourself a full manicure every week, but leave nails free of varnish for one day each week so that the air can get to them. Do not remove nail enamel more than once a week as the remover causes drying to the nail surface. If you want to change colour midweek paint a different colour on top of the existing one. Often you can produce some lovely colours by this method.

If your nails are not beautiful perhaps you would like to try false ones, but here again leave them off one day a week to allow your own nails to get some air. This avoids 'yellowing' of the nails.

Deportment and Being Photographed

Many ladies are not sure how to sit or how to look their best when they are being photographed. It takes practice to look elegant when walking, standing or sitting. Here are some suggestions.

Standing – Stand in front of a mirror and hold your tummy in. Tuck your bottom under and pull your shoulders back. Hold your head up and direct your eyes straight ahead. Now try to keep this position, but relax. See how good you look and how much slimmer you appear!

Walking – Imagine that as you walk you are being pulled by two strings which have been threaded through your hip bones. This is how models are taught to walk. Try to practise every day and soon it will become natural.

Often we stoop, particularly as we get older, and usually this is caused by pushing prams, push chairs, etc. It is most important to learn to straighten yourself as much as possible. Midriff bulges will disappear and you will look much younger. You can practise with a book on your head if you wish.

Sitting – Sit in front of a full-length mirror. There are three main sitting positions which are considered to be correct. Sit comfortably but upright in a chair.

Position 1 – Feet together but to one side (your big toe joint should fit into the arch of the outer foot). See Figure 1.

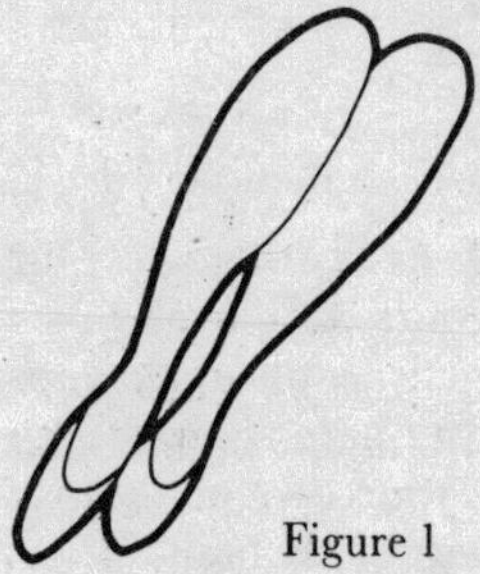

Figure 1

Position 2 – One foot tucked behind the other. Both feet placed to one side. See Figure 2.

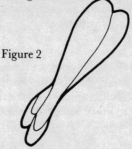

Figure 2

Position 3 – One leg over the other to one side, but knees level (one knee should not be further extended than the other). The legs should be in line with each other. See Figure 3.

Figure 3

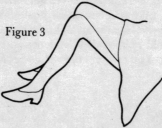

With all these positions, the legs should always be close together and in line with each other. Place your hands together on your lap, the opposite side to your feet.

Photography
General hints worth remembering when being photographed:

(a) Never stand straight on at the camera. Stand as we have discussed already (*Standing*), but lift one foot half a step backwards and turn the foot out slightly. Swivel the hips a few degrees (in the same direction as the back foot) and this will take inches off your hip width.

(b) Slip your handbag over one arm with your arm close to your waist. The other arm should be down by your side. If your bag is a clutch bag, hold it close to your waist, down by your side.

(c) If you can wear white next to your face it is very flattering.

(d) Remember that the person nearest to the camera will look a little larger than the one further away. If you are being photographed with someone who is smaller or slimmer, make sure that they are nearer to the camera!

Hygiene

Good grooming is essential to be attractive. A daily bath is desirable, but this alone will not keep you free from body odours. Everyone perspires – some more than others – and most perspiration evaporates quickly and is odourless. It is the stale perspiration that smells unpleasant, either on our bodies or on our clothes, and it can become stale within a few hours by being trapped under our arms and in various other places.

If we bathed several times a day in all the places where the perspiration gathers, and wore clean underwear and clothes, then the chances are that we would not smell. However, it is safer to use a deodorant, which helps to stop odour, although it doesn't prevent wetness. An anti-perspirant attempts to seal in the wetness, thus preventing perspiration in the first place, and therefore the ideal is a deodorant which combines both functions. The extra ingredients will keep you dry as well as odour-free.

If you suffer from excessive perspiration, try an extra-strong deodorant. Ask your chemist to advise you.

Often it is not the perspiration that smells, but the clothes we are wearing. Man-made fibres tend to make you sweat more and will not absorb the perspiration – in particular, polyester and nylon, but as these fabrics are easy to wash, there should be no excuse. Wool and cotton are more absorbent, but still hold the smell. Once perspiration gets into a natural-fibre garment it won't come out, so be careful.

Wear a man-made fibre garment for no more than 12 hours under normal circumstances. We perspire more when anxious or under any sort of stress. Beware of party dresses – we get warm at parties, so a dress should be worn preferably once, or twice at the most, before being cleaned.

It is a good idea to spray the palms of your hands with an anti-perspirant if you are about to attend an important function where you may be called upon to shake hands. Run cold water over your wrists for instant cooling down!

As well as applying a deodorant and anti-perspirant under your arms you may like to apply talc all over your body. This will absorb the moisture and will therefore save your clothes. Apply body lotion after a bath or shower. A complete change of underwear each day is also essential.

Beware of dark-coloured garments. Just because they don't look dirty it doesn't mean that they are fresh. You would only wear white once, so wear a dark-coloured garment no more than twice. Don't forget that things are much easier to wash when they are not too grubby. There will be no need to rub, and therefore the texture of the fabric will not be lost.

Experiment with deodorants – there are lots to choose from. Try to find one that really smells good. If you don't like a 'wet' one use a 'dry' one. It's a good idea to carry cologne sachets for a daytime freshen-up. Because we can become immune to one particular brand it is worthwhile changing your deodorant/anti-perspirant every few months.

Menstruation

If you suffer with period pains have a look at what you are eating. Avoid stodgy and sweet things. Do not drink too much alcohol. Vitamin C tablets might help, and also a little extra iron in tablet form could be taken.

If the pain continues, consult your doctor. If you feel tired and depressed it could be that you are anaemic.

Be extra careful with hygiene during your periods. Have lots of baths and be extravagant with talc, etc. Avoid using an intimate deodorant – these can do more harm than good and are unnecessary if proper attention is given to personal hygiene.

Take plenty of exercise during your period.

Feet

Wash frequently and for rough skin use a pumice stone, a 'foot scraper' or a branded 'rough-skin remover' cream. Cut toe nails straight across. There are special powders for cooling feet that perspire excessively and foot deodorants are also available.

Body Hair

Lip hair can be removed with a depilatory cream, but the instructions on the packet must be carefully followed. Alternatively, you may choose to have your lip waxed by a beautician, but *never* shave your face. Hair under the arms holds perspiration so always remove it, either with a lady's razor or a depilatory cream, or have it waxed. Hairs on the legs should be removed if they show, and the same depilatory cream could be used, but *do not shave* your legs. Waxing is more expensive, but it is a very efficient way of removing hair.

Teeth

Always clean your teeth regularly and carefully. See the dentist every six months. Try chewing a disclosing tablet (available from any chemist) as this will show up the parts of your teeth that are still unclean. If your breath smells use Gold Spot or Amplex. Be careful when you have eaten something strong like garlic or onions, or when you have been a long while without food. Cheese, coffee and milk can also make your breath smell unpleasant.

Hints on Good Grooming

1. Never rush. Don't frown. Keep a mirror in your kitchen to 'catch you out'
2. The best beauty treatment of all is fresh air, exercise and plenty of sleep
3. Try to keep up to date and try new styles – they might suit you. Try new hairstyles, but always give a new hairdresser two attempts before judging him, as he needs to get to know your hair
4. Always try to wear three colours. The third colour can be jewellery or a scarf, or even matching nail varnish and lipstick
5. Always be sure to check your back and front in the mirror before going out

7
Recognising a problem area

When you have to face up to the fact that your weight measuring belt is far too tight it is essential to take remedial action quickly. I certainly wouldn't suggest that you embark on a slimming diet, but just cut down by one third your normal day's consumption of food and drink or alternatively select from the special menus on pages 124–9.

The simple solution to any weight problem is to observe the following recommendations.

Follow your normal everyday eating plan but:
1. Reduce the amount of fat
2. Reduce the amount of sugar
3. Avoid fried foods
4. Restrict your consumption of milk to ¼ pint (150ml)
5. Increase your level of physical activity
6. Use a smaller plate at every meal
7. Reduce your alcoholic consumption by a third

It is always helpful to use low-calorie substitute foods during this comparatively short period such as:

1. St Ivel Gold low-fat spread instead of butter or margarine
2. Hermesetas Gold artificial sweetener (it really doesn't leave an aftertaste)
3. Always grill rather than fry and remove any fat from meat *before* you cook it
4. Skimmed milk instead of whole milk
5. There are some splendid recipes for delicious drinks on pages 120–24.

Alternatively, if you can afford it, why not treat yourself to a visit to a health resort for a holiday, or go to some kind of activity holiday either for a week or just for a weekend.

Let us look at health farms first.

At the top end of the market there is Champneys at Tring in Hertfordshire. The house and grounds are spectacular and the treatment areas and leisure facilities are of the highest standard. I recently spent a week there and found the experience fascinating, but quite hard work! The different classes held each day ranged from dance exercise to yoga and relaxation. There was also a gym for anyone who wanted a very hard workout, and evening classes teaching a wide variety of subjects including dancing, painting, flower arranging and the art of positive thinking. We were also able to watch the head chef demonstrating the preparation of a splendid selection of recipes for low-calorie dishes. Tennis courts and delightful country walks completed the feeling of 'getting away from it all'!

The price of your stay will vary according to your choice of bedroom, and really depends on how much you are prepared to pay. It is expensive, but *how* expensive is totally dependent upon your personal means. Included in the price is a personal consultation with a qualified nurse who will advise you on the most beneficial treatments to suit your state of health. If necessary she will suggest you have a consultation with the visiting doctor. You will also have the opportunity to meet the resident dietician who will advise you about diet and record your weight loss progress. Every day you will be given a massage and a heat treatment – either a sauna, steam cabinet or a spa bath. Other beauty treatments are available too, but these will cost you extra.

There are two dining rooms – the light diet and the main dining room. In the light diet room only very low-calorie dishes are served and the daily intake is around 500. In the main dining room there is a choice between the menu of the day or an attractively displayed cold buffet. All dishes were delicious, oozing with goodness and perfectly adequate, but I did feel that there was a definite lack of supervision here, as you could eat as much as you liked even though you were supposed to be restricting your intake. The lounge bar offered delicious low-calorie drinks during most of the day – an education in itself!

Weight losses enjoyed by many guests were impressive, but some were disappointed at having lost only a pound or two (½–1 kilo). However, the treatments and exercise sessions certainly help you become fitter and tone the body into a much more acceptable shape, and you certainly won't become bored during your stay. In fact, my only criticism would be that there is too much to do! As I didn't want to miss anything I found it difficult to relax.

The directors who are responsible for the overall appearance and performance of this luxury health resort are Allan and Tanya Wheway, and I must say they do an excellent job. I was sorry not to see more of Mrs Wheway during my stay, because when I attended a dinner at a later date at which she was the guest speaker, I realised how inspiring she is. Her talk was most interesting and I came away feeling uplifted. She certainly is a remarkable lady and I wish her the very best of luck in her determined efforts to help her guests towards a happier and healthier life.

To sum up, if you can afford it, Champneys offers the height of luxury combined with expert help. It may well help you to lose those few pounds that have crept on, but you need to resolve that you will be moderate in your eating while you are there, and to maintain the healthy eating pattern when you return home. If you cannot justify the expense for a whole week, Champneys take day guests offering a variety of treatments at fairly moderate prices.

Further details of Champneys at Tring can be obtained by writing to General Enquiries, Champneys at Tring, Tring, Hertfordshire or telephoning Berkhamsted 3351.

If you feel like a complete rest in a very relaxed environment at a very low cost I would suggest you visit Tyringham Clinic in Buckinghamshire. It is a charitable organisation so the tariff is very moderate and you don't have to pay VAT. The cost depends on the type of room you choose – sharing a room with five or six others means that the rate is extremely low, but it could double if you wanted a single room with full facilities. However, the treatments are the same no matter which room you choose.

Tyringham is not a typical health resort. It combines medical treatment with health tuition, based on naturopathic medicine and vegetarian food, and aims to treat patients with conditions ranging from arthritis to obesity. You are therefore a patient, not a guest. Facilities available include the usual sauna, steam bath and massage, but extend far beyond these to acupuncture and osteopathy. Treatments to improve circulation and respiration take high priority. All treatments as prescribed are included in your room rate, and only blood tests or necessary medication incur extra charges.

The staff at Tyringham are fully trained and totally dedicated to their cause. They are extremely friendly at all times, as are the patients. There is a magical atmosphere about the place, and when I have spent time there I have come away feeling relaxed, looking younger and able to cope with anything! In fact, Tyringham made such a deep impression on me that it played a major part in encouraging me to study yoga and slimming techniques in considerable depth.

Most patients are requested to fast for a few days in order to cleanse their system and eliminate toxins. They are then introduced to a very light diet followed by a normal but delicious vegetarian diet. Portions are set out so there is no chance of cheating! Lemon and honey or a variety of fruit juices are the main drinks offered during the day, but every afternoon you are allowed a cup of tea. Many varieties are available from which to choose. It is strange to experience the extreme pleasure of that one drink when normally we take such beverages for granted several times a day.

Weight losses are usually satisfactory ranging from 3 to 10 pounds (1·5 to 4·5 kilos) per week. Providing you eat sensibly when returning home the weight shouldn't return, particularly as advice is given on departure on how to 'keep up the good work'.

The house and grounds of Tyringham Clinic are delightful, set in acres and acres of beautiful countryside. When I am there I refuse to watch television, read newspapers or even venture to the nearby villages. It is almost like a retreat to me and I feel it is very beneficial. I recently returned to Tyringham after some years. Whilst some staff had changed, the atmosphere was as superb as ever, and I intend to return again soon to enjoy the pure qualities of this special establishment.

Daily activities include some form of exercise session in the gym or yoga, or relaxation plus various water treatments from spa baths to sitz baths (you sit in a divided bath with warm water in one end and cold in the other and after a few minutes you are asked to change round!). Alternatively, you may be prescribed a Scottish douche, where hot and cold water are sprayed alternately on your back after sea salt has been rubbed all over you. Your skin feels terrific and you certainly feel exhilarated. There are also saunas, sunbeds and a whirlpool to enjoy.

You cannot 'buy' extra treatments. You are told which ones are most suited to you and your day's treatment list is left by your bedroom door each night. However, extensive leisure facilities, including a swimming pool, tennis courts, table tennis and much more, are available for use at no extra cost.

There is time to relax and chat with other guests, but there is also a certain amount of necessary discipline. Tyringham also offers a single day 'out-patient' facility where you can enjoy various treatments prescribed by your consultant. If you would like to find out more about Tyringham write to Tyringham Naturopathic Clinic,

Tyringham, Newport Pagnell, Buckinghamshire or telephone Newport Pagnell 610450.

If a week away is inconvenient you could try a Holiday Inn Successful Slimming Health and Beauty Weekender. I felt very honoured to be asked by Holiday Inns if I would design a programme of activities and run the weekenders at most of their inns throughout the United Kingdom. Because the first series of five held in 1983/4 proved so popular, it was decided to organise a series of seven during the latter part of 1984 and in early 1985. Reasonably priced, the accommodation and facilities are of the highest standard and the atmosphere at all the Holiday Inns at which I have stayed is pleasant and very relaxed. The Weekenders commence on a Friday afternoon when guests are welcome to have a swim and a sauna and use the gym equipment available at all of their hotels. In the evening there is a welcome cocktail party (slimmer's cocktails, of course) followed by dinner, and then a make-up demonstration by one of Boots' top beauty therapists where everyone receives a sample of something from the Boots No. 7 range.

Saturday starts with a healthy but calorie-counted breakfast followed by a talk on successful slimming. Then it is time for a Slimobility session and after a mid-morning slimmers' cocktail some pool exercises. After lunch guests are free to have a sauna, a sunbed treatment and a swim, and also use the gym equipment. Then there's an optional 'Making the most of yourself' lecture, and finally Saturday's activities are rounded off later in the afternoon with a yoga and deep relaxation session. Dinner is served early in the evening so anyone wishing to visit the theatre may do so, or alternatively they can join in the dinner dance within the hotel.

On Sunday morning after breakfast there is another talk, where the benefits of being slim and the purpose of exercise are explained. The guests then divide into groups of elementary and advanced students. The advanced students go for a jog in the local park and then participate in a very energetic Slimobility session. Meanwhile the less fit students enjoy a gentle Slimobility session followed by a brisk walk outside the hotel.

After lunch guests are encouraged to stay so that they can continue enjoying the excellent leisure facilities available in the hotel until 4 p.m.

All the meals are calorie counted, and whilst you have to restrict yourself at breakfast and lunchtimes because the meals are available from a buffet, the evening meal is served in appropriately sized portions. Because the food is always so delicious I doubt whether many guests actually lose weight during their Weekenders, but I do know they enjoy themselves and feel better for the break away from their families. I certainly thoroughly enjoy running the Weekenders and I hope they will continue for many more years to come. For further details write to Jane Brooks, Executive Offices, Holiday Inns, Slough, Bucks or telephone Slough 44255.

Another kind of activity holiday was organised in 1984 by Swinards Coach Tours. It included seven nights at a luxury hotel in the beautiful resort of Lech in Austria at a very low cost indeed. It is anticipated that similar holidays will be available from 1985 onwards.

I was delighted to be invited to supervise the activity holidays and because we were away for a week the programme of the activities was less intense than on the Weekenders. Swimming in the pool, treasure hunts, Slimobility sessions in the local gym, saunas and excursions to nearby towns and also to Italy, made the holidays particularly interesting. Tennis or squash facilities were also available to guests. The amount of activity undertaken was completely optional and guests were given the alternative of just lazing around in the sun if they preferred. The scenery was breathtaking and the air so pure we all felt wonderful at the end of the week. Weight losses were spectacular too, with some guests shedding as much as 6 to 8 pounds (3 to 4 kilos).

If you would like to know more about these activity

holidays write to Swinards, Ashford, Kent or telephone Ashford 36061.

No matter which idea appeals to you most, I am *certain* you will enjoy yourself.

8
The occasional downfall

Occasionally we find we have gained a few pounds, perhaps after visiting a favourite aunty who makes the most glorious scones, or entertaining guests for the weekend. Because you want to make them feel welcome you bake cakes, cook exotic dishes and buy many extra treats. But who eats the left-overs when they go home? The last bit of trifle? The apple pie? 'It's *such* a shame to waste them . . .'

Try and be sensible when you find yourself caught in situations like these. Don't have second helpings. Eat smaller portions and drink lots of cups of tea. You will soon feel satisfied.

However, this chapter gives advice on how to deal with yourself when you have not had small portions at all! You've made a real pig of yourself and you know you must have gained weight – it feels like loads of weight too! You think you look terribly fat when in actual fact most of your overindulgence is still being stored around your digestive organs. Because the body has not been given a chance to process it all, most of the excess has not in fact turned to fat yet, but it will if you don't do something about it soon!

I always tell my slimmers after they have gorged themselves beyond all reason at Christmastime that if they are really good for the following week most of the excess will disappear as quickly as it arrived; and it certainly does disappear. As much as 7 pounds (3 kilos) of quickly gained weight can be lost in a week by cutting right down – not starving of course – but being very sensible over what food is chosen.

It is important to realise what our bodies actually need to be healthy. Beyond the basic requirements additional food in moderation can be included to enhance the variety of one's daily diet. When we have been overindulgent, all that is necessary is to stick to only the basic nutritional necessities.

These are as follows:

PER DAY
4–6oz/100–150g protein foods (i.e., moderate helpings of meat, fish, eggs or cheese)
3 pieces fresh fruit (any type)
6oz/150g fresh or frozen vegetables (any kind)
¼ pint/150ml fresh milk or ½ pint/300ml skimmed
3oz (75g) cereal or grain foods (cereals, bread, rice, pasta, etc.)
¼oz/7g fat in any form or ½oz/15g low-fat spread
You may drink as much fresh or bottled water (e.g., Ashbourne or Perrier) or low-calorie drinks as you wish.

If you follow these simple guidelines for approximately seven days after gaining some weight I am sure you will lose *all* your excess.

Thereafter attempt to maintain your weight by following these recommended quantities but gradually increase them again, combining into your diet a few carefully chosen treats, so that you may return to normal healthy eating without gaining an ounce.

At the same time as trying to lose your excess poundage, why not increase your energy output too.

9
Exercise machines

I am often asked my opinion of exercise equipment to be used at home. Slimmers seem to think that an exercise bicycle will be the answer to everything. Unfortunately it won't, but used regularly and properly, along with other keep-fit gadgets, it *can* help to keep you looking better as well as helping to maintain or even increase your metabolic rate.

Given below is a list of the equipment I have tried together with my unbiased opinion:

Exercise Bicycle

Used daily this can certainly help to tone up the legs and bottom, and benefit the feet and ankles. There is also a small increase in stamina. Cycling outside is a totally different activity. It will certainly build up stamina as well as strengthening the legs a great deal. The reason for the greater benefit is:

1. You will be breathing fresh air
2. The activity will be more interesting as the scenery will be constantly changing
3. You will find outdoor cycling more energetic because you will be going uphill at times and generally concentrating much harder
4. When you have cycled a few miles you will really feel you have achieved something

Rowing Machine

If I were to choose between an exercise bicycle or a rowing machine I would definitely go for the latter. A rowing machine utilises so many more muscles in just one complete stroke: arms, tummy, buttocks, back, legs, ankles and feet. It is a great all-round toner.

Multi-Gym

This is an arrangement of bars and weights cleverly designed to enable you to exercise every part of your body whether for strength, stamina or suppleness. However, as with any equipment that is so extensive in its benefits, it is expensive. Also it is fairly large and you would need not only sufficient room but also a good strong floor on which to place it!

Bar with Weights

Inexpensive and easy to use, a bar with additional weights is available in men's and women's sizes. Used properly they can strengthen your muscles and improve your body shape. Most of the benefits will be to the arms, chest and back, but they can be used over the ankles to strengthen the legs. There is no need to be frightened of building a body like Mr Universe if you are a woman. Women really are made quite differently and a build-up of muscle to equal his is impossible.

Dum-bells

The benefits are much the same as for a weight bar except that because they are smaller they can be used in both hands and operated quite separately. They can be fun if used with music accompanying your exercises, as can a bar and weights.

Bench

A small padded bench is a superb piece of equipment. You can lie upward or downward, exercise your legs while suspended in the air, and exercise your arms too. By tucking your feet under the end bar you can do sit-ups easily.

Bullworker

This is a marvellous piece of equipment which is extremely versatile. Bodybuilding is its main purpose, and I have seen amazing results achieved in only six weeks of regular and proper use. Bullworkers are sensibly priced and can be hidden away with ease. A comprehensive instruction booklet comes with them, too.

Door Exercisers

This is a very inexpensive piece of equipment which basically consists of strong elastic ropes (rather like the expanding clip-on luggage holders used on roofracks). These are positioned over a door knob, and by using your arms and legs you can get a reasonable toning effect. I found the exercise boring, however, and could not persevere.

Slendertone
(or similar passive exercise machines)

A passive exercise machine exercises muscles while you lie on a couch or bed. A portable machine running on batteries is available, or a larger electrically powered 'salon' model. Both come supplied with full instructions for correct usage.

The portable machine consists of an operating unit plus eight plastic-covered wires which in turn are connected to round rubber pads. The pads are placed at strategic points on your body (depending on which part you wish to tone), and are held in place with wide elasticated bands. The machine works on the body by activating the muscles you wish to tone without physical movement. Your legs may feel like they have walked 30 miles at the end of your 40-minute session, but you won't have sore feet or feel at all tired!

This all sounds too good to be true, but there are certain disadvantages. The machines are not cheap, and are very time consuming. They are extremely inconvenient if someone calls unexpectedly at your door!

No passive exercise machine will eliminate fat. You can only do that by reducing your energy input by calorie cutting and increasing your energy output by taking *real* exercise. However, they can help on your muscle shape and they will certainly make your long-lost muscles come back to life, so if for any reason you can't take normal exercise a machine could be invaluable to you. For some people they work very well, but not everyone can tolerate the strange sensation given out by some of these machines.

Vibrating Belts

These consist of a base on which you stand, with a motor placed at the top of a column in front of you. Attached to this is a wide belt which you place around the parts of your body you wish to tone. After switching on, very fast vibrations are felt through the belt. Used regularly it might help to lessen the volume of excesses, but the vibrations caused me to itch like crazy. Try one out before you buy it; they are very boring to use.

To Sum Up

Before buying new exercise equipment, remember that a lot of people have already bought it and found they hadn't the patience to use it regularly enough to be effective. Why not place an advertisement in your local newspaper. I bought all my equipment that way and always paid less than half price, sometimes only 25 per cent of the original cost.

Don't allow yourself to fall into the trap of buying a new 'wonder gadget' only to find that after a week/month it goes into the loft. Whatever machine or gadget you buy, it will only have a chance of helping you if you use it *very regularly*. Once a week will not produce any benefit at all.

So, don't let yours be the equipment up for sale again in six months! Let it be your beautifully toned-up body that friends wish was theirs, not your unused rowing machine!

At the end of the day, a brisk walk will do as much if not more to improve your figure, as well as enabling you to breath in fresh air and enjoy the view. Your dog or children would prefer it too!

10
Recipes

Here are some delicious recipes which will hopefully become part of your normal way of eating. Because they are lower in calories than many other recipes does not mean they cannot taste good; these will taste even better.

You will notice that some products have been included in certain recipes. These are designed to reduce the calorie content, and in my opinion they are nutritionally sound. Alternative products of your choice may be used if preferred providing the calorie content is similar.

Within this chapter are offered complete menus, drinks, snacks and desserts.

Calorie-counted Drinks

Alcoholic

Planter's Punch
Serves 10 69 calories per serving

½ pint/300ml dark rum
1 tablespoon lemon juice
1 pint/600ml orange squash
chopped orange
chopped kiwi fruit
crushed ice (optional)

1 teaspoon sugar
Ashbourne natural sparkling
 water

Mix rum, lemon juice, orange squash, chopped orange, kiwi fruit and sugar together in large jug. Chill well. Transfer into thermos flask, with crushed ice if liked, and top with Ashbourne natural sparkling water.

Cool Cup
Serves 8 57 calories per serving

4 tablespoons blackcurrant
  cordial
½ bottle white wine (chilled)
1 pint/600ml Ashbourne
  natural sparkling water
  (chilled)

crushed ice
fresh mint

Pour the blackcurrant cordial into a large jug. Add chilled white wine, Ashbourne natural sparkling water, crushed ice and sprigs of mint. Transfer into thermos flasks to keep cool.

Tropical Sunset
Serves 1 41 calories per serving

1fl oz/25ml vodka
1fl oz/25ml tomato juice
1fl oz/25ml Ashbourne
  natural sparkling water
slice of lemon

Mix together vodka and tomato juice. Top with Ashbourne natural sparkling water. Garnish with a slice of lemon.

Lime Cocktail Cooler
Serves 1 135 calories per serving

½fl oz/12ml lime juice
ice
1fl oz/25ml vodka
1fl oz/25ml Martini
Ashbourne natural sparkling
  water (chilled)
slices of fresh lime

Pour lime over ice into a tall glass. Add vodka and Martini, and top up with chilled Ashbourne natural sparkling water. Add slices of fresh lime.

Ashbourne Royale
Serves 1 110 calories per serving

2fl oz/50ml champagne
1fl oz/25ml gin
drops of lemon juice
1 teaspoon sugar

crushed ice
Ashbourne natural sparkling
 water

Pour ingredients over crushed ice and top with Ashbourne natural sparkling water.

Non-Alcoholic

St Clement's
Serves 1 40 calories per serving

1 bottle slimline bitter lemon
4fl oz/100ml fresh orange
 juice
ice

slice of lemon
slice of orange
fresh mint

Mix the ingredients together, add ice and garnish with a slice of lemon and orange and a mint leaf.

Grapefruit Fizz
Serves 1 30 calories per serving

1 bottle slimline tonic
4fl oz/100ml fresh
 unsweetened grapefruit
 juice

ice
slice of lemon

Mix the ingredients together and serve with ice and a slice of lemon.

Ashbourne Chiller
Calorie-free

Ashbourne natural sparkling
 water (chilled)

ice
slice of lemon

Pour chilled Ashbourne natural sparkling water over ice into a tumbler and top with a slice of lemon. (To keep cool store refrigerated bottled water in an ice box.)

Cutie Fruitie
Serves 6 64 calories per serving

17fl oz/425ml Libby's Orange
  'C'
9fl oz/225ml Libby's
  Pineapple 'C'
9fl oz/225ml Libby's Apple
  'C'

chopped orange
fresh mint
crushed ice

Mix all ingredients together and chill well. To serve decorate with fresh fruit, a sprig of mint and a drinking straw.

Sundowner
Serves 1 52 calories per serving

½ glass unsweetened orange
  juice
2 tablespoons lemon juice
1 tablespoon lime cordial

1 teaspoon grenadine
Ashbourne natural sparkling
  water
ice

Put the first three ingredients in a cocktail shaker or screw-top jar and shake well. Pour grenadine into glass, add contents of shaker and top up with Ashbourne natural sparkling water and ice.

Orange Yogurt Surprise
Serves 3 52 calories per serving

2 oranges
4 tablespoons natural yoghurt
6 drops liquid sweetener

¾ pint/450ml Ashbourne
  natural sparkling water
  (chilled)
ice

Cut three slices from one orange, then squeeze the juice from the rest of the orange into a small bowl together with the juice from the second orange. Beat the yoghurt and the sweetener into the orange juice. Whisk in the chilled Ashbourne natural sparkling water. Place some ice cubes into three goblet glasses and add the orange drink. Decorate with slices of orange.

123

Cucumber Snow
Serves 2 66 calories per serving

4oz/100g cucumber
8oz/100g natural yoghurt
½ teaspoon salt
1 small clove garlic

½ pint/300ml Ashbourne
  natural sparkling water
  (chilled)

Peel and slice the cucumber reserving four slices for garnishing. Place the cucumber into a blender and add the yoghurt, salt and peeled clove of garlic. Blend until smooth. Pour into two tumblers and top up with Ashbourne natural sparkling water. Decorate with cucumber slices.

Chocolate Cascade
Serves 4 115 calories per serving

4 scoops chocolate ice cream
few drops blackcurrant
  flavouring

1 pint/600ml Ashbourne
  natural sparkling water
1 tablespoon cocoa powder

Spoon the chocolate ice cream into four sundae glasses until they are all about one third full. Top up with Ashbourne natural sparkling water, then sprinkle the foamy heads with cocoa powder.

Menus

The following menus were created by some of our members in Northern Ireland. A competition was held to find the tastiest low-cost, low-calorie menu. Shirley Whiteside won first prize (menu 1), Edilia Pardolfi won second prize (menu 2), and Maria Pardolfi came third (menu 3).

The Pardolfi family had a great sense of humour, producing dishes which included the names of the company trademark (SSAGG), their class lecturer Patience (*Patience Cocktail*), renown for her bubbly personality (*Bubbling Peach*), and her husband called Ivor (*Ivor Steak*)! The runners-up, Diana Haines and Ruth Pieut, produced menus 4 and 5 respectively.

Low-Calorie Menus

All dishes serve 2, and calorie counts include one glass of wine per person

Menu 1

WINE
Lutomer Riesling (medium dry)

STARTER
59 calories per portion

2 oranges
½ red-skinned eating apple, chopped

1 stick celery, chopped
1 tablespoon cucumber, chopped

Cut top of oranges and scoop out centre. Scallop edges of oranges. Cut up flesh and mix with all other ingredients. Divide mixture in two and spoon back into orange cups ready to serve.

MAIN COURSE
362 calories per portion

1 large onion, chopped
2 chicken pieces (preferably thighs)
1 carrot, sliced
1 tablespoon mixed green/red peppers, chopped

4oz/100g mushrooms, sliced
¼ pint/150ml chicken stock
dash cider
2 medium-sized potatoes, baked

Place the onion in a casserole dish and half cover with water. Simmer slightly to soften onions. Add chicken pieces and surround with carrot, peppers, and mushrooms. Pour in chicken stock and cider, and season to taste. Cover tightly and cook in medium hot oven for 1 hour. Serve hot from casserole with baked potato.

DESSERT
100 calories per portion

3 tablespoons stewed rhubarb sweetened with saccharine to taste

2 small cartons natural low-fat yoghurt
nuts, finely chopped
two cherries

Using cold stewed rhubarb, mix thoroughly with yoghurt and divide between two dishes. Sprinkle with nuts and place cherry on top of each dish to decorate.

Menu 2

WINE
Colman's French white

MOUTHWATERING CRAB
44 calories per portion

1 medium tomato	2 lettuce leaves
2oz/50g cucumber	½ lemon
2oz/50g crab (fresh or tinned)	

Chop tomato, cucumber, crab and lettuce into small pieces. Mix together and squeeze the juice of half a lemon over. Serve in 2 glasses.

CHICKEN SSAGG
215 calories per portion

2 6oz/150g pieces of chicken	1 small onion, chopped
½ small packet of frozen peas	½ pint/300ml water
small tin peeled tomatoes	

Place the two pieces of chicken in an oven dish. Add the onion, peas and tomato, and season to taste. Add the water. Bake in oven (375°F, 190°C, Gas Mark 5) for 1½ hours.

STRAWBERRY ZEST
30 calories per portion

1 8oz/200g basket
   strawberries
juice of ½ lemon
juice of ½ orange

Rub strawberries through a sieve to obtain a thick liquid. Add the lemon and orange juice. Leave in freezer for 2 hours. Serve in a glass.

Menu 3

Colman's French red

PATIENCE COCKTAIL
35 calories per portion

¼ medium-sized onion,
  chopped
3 large iceberg lettuce leaves,
  chopped
1 tomato, chopped

5 slices cucumber, chopped
2oz/50g prawns
1 teaspoon vegetable oil
juice of ½ lemon
salt and black pepper

Mix all the ingredients together and toss. Serve in a glass.

IVOR STEAK
312 calories per portion

1½ teaspoons butter
2 garlic cloves, chopped
½ can peeled tomatoes,
  chopped
2 4oz/100g sirloin steaks

salt
1 teaspoon oregano
8oz/200g cauliflower
8oz/200g carrots

Heat the butter and garlic in a frying pan until golden brown. Add tomatoes, steaks, salt and oregano. Cook as required. Make sure the sauce is thick and not watery. If too dry add a little water. Serve with boiled cauliflower and carrots.

BUBBLING PEACH
58 calories per portion

2 fresh peaches
2 large scoops orange sorbet
1 bottle Babycham

Peel and slice the peaches. Place on the bottom of 2 champagne glasses. Add 1 scoop of sorbet to each glass. Pour ½ bottle of Babycham on each glass. Serve chilled.

Menu 4

STARTER
44 calories per portion

6oz/150g slice of melon
2 thin slices smoked Ardennes
   ham

Cut melon in half and replace on skin. Garnish with ham.

MAIN COURSE
526 calories per portion

6oz/150g rainbow trout
2 small potatoes, baked
2oz/50g sweetcorn, tinned
2oz/50g French beans
1 teaspoon cinnamon
2oz/50g celery
1oz/25g Edam cheese
2 slices lemon

1 teaspoon fresh parsley,
   chopped
1 small tomato, sliced

Grill the trout for 10 minutes. Cut the baked potatoes in half and scoop out the contents. Mix with sweetcorn and return to the jackets. Boil the French beans until tender and sprinkle with cinnamon. Braise the celery and cover with melted Edam. Garnish with the lemon, parsley and tomato.

DESSERT
192 calories per portion

2 medium-sized cooking
   apples
2oz/50g ice cream
½oz/15g honey

Wash and core the apples and bake in a moderately hot oven (375°F, 190°C, Gas Mark 5) for approximately 30 minutes. Fill the centre of each apple with ice cream and top with honey.

Menu 5
WINE
Piesporter

GRAPEFRUIT WITH COTTAGE CHEESE
80 calories per portion

1 large grapefruit
3oz/75g cottage cheese
1 teaspoon fresh parsley,
  chopped

Divide the grapefruit in two and top with cottage cheese.
Garnish with parsley.

BREAST OF CHICKEN WITH ORANGE AND TARRAGON
340 calories per portion

2 6oz/150g chicken breasts   2 courgettes, finely chopped
  (skin removed)   2 tomatoes, finely chopped
4fl oz/100ml fresh orange   8oz/200g broccoli
  juice   1 teaspoon basil
1 teaspoon tarragon   1 teaspoon oregano

Place the chicken breasts in a shallow dish together with
the orange juice and sprinkle with tarragon. Cover with a
lid and bake in a moderately hot oven (375°F, 190°C, Gas
Mark 5) for 35 minutes. Mix the courgette and tomato
and season with basil and oregano. Serve together with
the broccoli, which should be cooked until tender.

FRESH FRUIT SALAD
125 calories per portion

1 kiwi, sliced   1oz/25g black grapes
1 apple, sliced   1oz/25g green grapes
1 orange, divided into   1 pear, sliced
  segments   4fl oz/100ml fresh orange
1 peach, sliced   juice

Mix together the ingredients listed above and serve in a
long glass.

Individual dishes

Main Courses

Ratatouille Stuffed Pancakes
Serves 6 315 calories per portion

PANCAKE BATTER

4oz/100g plain flour	1 large can Nestlé Tip Top
1 egg	butter or lard for frying

FILLING

2oz/50g butter	½ pint/300ml tomato juice
1 large onion, sliced	salt
1 small red pepper, diced	freshly ground black pepper
1 clove garlic, crushed	1oz/25g butter
1 small aubergine, diced	4oz/100g Cheddar cheese,
4 small courgettes, sliced	grated
2 bay leaves	chopped parsley for garnish

Preheat the oven to 350°F, 180°C, Gas Mark 4.

To make the batter, place the flour in a bowl and make a well in the centre. Add the egg and gradually beat in the Tip Top until smooth.

Heat a knob of butter or lard in a small frying pan, ensuring it coats the base of the pan. Pour in enough batter to cover the base of the pan thinly, and cook for 3 minutes or until golden brown. Toss or turn and cook the remaining side until golden. Repeat to make 12 pancakes. Stack the pancakes on a plate, layered with greaseproof paper. Cover and keep warm.

To make the filling, melt the butter in a large frying pan. Add the onion, red pepper, garlic and aubergine, and fry, stirring until just beginning to soften. Add the courgettes and cook for a further two minutes. Stir in the bay leaves, tomato juice and season well. Cover and cook for a further 15 minutes or until the vegetables are just tender. Remove the bay leaves.

Spoon 2 spoonfuls of the ratatouille mixture on to each pancake, fold in the sides and roll up.

Melt the butter in a shallow ovenproof dish. Arrange the pancakes in the base. Sprinkle with cheese and place in the oven for 10 to 15 minutes until they are heated through and the cheese has melted. Garnish with the chopped parsley.

Spinach Quiche
Serves 6 395 calories per portion

6oz/150g shortcrust pastry
1 small onion, sliced
1oz/25g butter
8oz/200g frozen spinach, thawed
3oz/75g mature English Cheddar

3 eggs
1 large can Nestlé Tip Top
salt
freshly ground black pepper
1 tablespoon grated Parmesan cheese

Preheat the oven to 400°F, 200°C, Gas Mark 6. Roll out the pastry and use to line a 9-inch flan ring or dish. Fry the onion in the butter until soft then add the spinach and cook for a further 2 minutes. Arrange in the base of the pastry case. Sprinkle with Cheddar cheese. Beat together the Tip Top and eggs and season well. Pour the mixture over the spinach and cheese. Sprinkle with Parmesan. Place in the oven for 30 to 40 minutes until set and golden brown.

Serve with a crisp green salad.

Bread and Cheese Pudding
Serves 4 443 calories per portion

6 slices wholemeal bread
made mustard
6oz/150g mature English Cheddar
1 large can Nestlé Tip Top

¼ pint/150ml water
3 eggs beaten
1 teaspoon salt
freshly ground black pepper

Preheat the oven to 350°F, 180°C, Gas Mark 4.

Spread the bread slices generously on one side with the mustard, then cut each slice into triangles.

Arrange a layer of the bread in the bottom of a buttered shallow ovenproof dish. Sprinkle over a layer of cheese. Repeat until all the bread and cheese have been used, finishing with a layer of cheese.

Beat together the Tip Top, water and eggs. Season well with the salt and pepper. Pour on to the bread and cheese. Cook in the oven for about 30 minutes until set and golden brown. Serve with a crisp salad

Tip Top Yoghurt
515 calories

1 large can Nestlé Tip Top
1 teaspoon natural yoghurt

Fill a wide-mouthed thermos flask with boiling water and leave for a few minutes. Meanwhile, warm the Tip Top in a saucepan. Empty the thermos flask and add the yoghurt. Pour in a little of the heated Tip Top, mix until smooth, then add the rest. Screw on the thermos lid and leave for a minimum of 6 hours or preferably overnight. Then remove the yoghurt from the flask and chill well before using. This recipe makes ¾ pint/450ml of creamy yoghurt which is low in cholesterol and animal fats.

Iced Orange Yoghurt Shake
Serves 2 132 calories per portion

½ pint/300ml unsweetened
   orange juice
¼ pint/150ml Tip Top
   yoghurt
4 ice cubes

Place all the ingredients in a food blender and liquidise until smooth.
Variations:
grapefruit, pineapple or tomato juice can be used instead of orange juice.

Chilled Tomato Yoghurt Soup
Serves 4 110 calories per portion

½ pint/300ml Tip Top
  yoghurt (see page 132)
1 pint/600ml tomato juice
1 tablespoon Worcestershire
  sauce

salt
pepper
½ green pepper, diced

Whisk together the Tip Top yoghurt and tomato juice. Add the Worcestershire sauce and season to taste. Pour into individual soup bowls and chill well. Just before serving garnish with the green pepper.

Minted Cucumber and Yoghurt Salad
Serves 4 45 calories per portion

1 medium-sized cucumber
¼ pint/150ml Tip Top
  yoghurt
1 tablespoon lemon juice

2 teaspoons mint, chopped
salt
freshly ground black pepper

With a potato peeler remove the cucumber skin, then slice the cucumber into ⅛-inch slices. Arrange overlapping on a serving dish.

Mix together the Tip Top yoghurt, lemon juice and mint and season to taste with the salt and pepper. Pour in the centre of the cucumber slices.

Variations: For a tomato salad substitute fresh basil for the mint and for a green salad substitute chopped fennel and parsley.

Winter Salad
Serves 1 60 calories per portion

1 small tomato
1 small onion, preferably
  Spanish
1 carrot
3oz/75g raw white cabbage
¼ green or red pepper
few sprigs raw cauliflower

1 raw mushroom, chopped
pinch of parsley, marjoram
  and chervil
salt and freshly ground
  pepper
juice of ¼ lemon
1 tablespoon cider vinegar

Slice the tomato and finely shred the onion, carrot, cabbage and green or red pepper. Break the cauliflower sprigs into tiny florets. Combine all the vegetables, including the chopped mushroom, and add the herbs and seasonings. Toss in a large bowl with the lemon juice and cider vinegar. Cover and leave in the refrigerator to marinate, preferably for 1½ hours or more.

Slimline Jelly
Serves 4 12 calories per portion

½oz/15g gelatine
  (1 envelope)
1 pint/600ml cold water
2oz/50g blackberries (fresh or
  frozen) or similar fruit

10 artificial sweetener tablets
squeeze of lemon juice

Soak the gelatine in a little of the water in a pan, off the heat. Place the fruit and artificial sweetener in another pan with ¼ pint/150ml of the water and simmer gently until the fruit is cooked and the liquid is a good colour. Add the lemon juice and the remaining water.

Meanwhile, gently heat the gelatine until dissolved. Pour the cooked fruit on to the gelatine liquid and stir well. Place in four individual moulds or dishes, making sure that the fruit is distributed evenly.

Serve with 2 tablespoons top of the milk (16 calories) or 1 tablespoon whipping cream (25 calories).

Apricot Delight
Serves 6 99 calories per portion

8oz/200g dried apricots
2 teaspoons powdered
  gelatine
2 tablespoons water

1 small can Nestlé Tip Top
1 teaspoon lemon juice
lemon slices for decoration

Soak the apricots in a large bowl overnight.

Dissolve the gelatine in the water by placing it in a small bowl over a saucepan of hot water.

Place the apricots and their liquid (made up to ¾ pint/450ml with water), gelatine and Tip Top in a blender or food processor. Blend until smooth. Stir in the lemon juice. Spoon into 6 individual glasses and decorate with the twists of lemon.

Raspberry and Almond Junket
Serves 4 179 calories per portion

1oz/25g powdered gelatine	½ teaspoon almond essence
4 tablespoons castor sugar	8oz/200g raspberries (fresh or
1 small can Nestlé Tip Top	frozen)
1 pint/600ml water	

Put the gelatine, sugar, Tip Top and water in a saucepan. Place over a low heat until the gelatine dissolves. Add the almond essence and pour into a bowl. Allow to cool. Refrigerate for 3 hours or until set.

Cut the junket into cubes and place in individual dishes. Spoon over the raspberries with any juice.

11
Questions and answers

I am often asked various questions with particular regard to gaining weight. I take this opportunity to answer a few of them.

Q. *I am having a baby in 7 months' time. I dread regaining all the weight that I have lost. What can I do?*
A. First of all forget about eating for two; your body will tell you when it is really hungry. Forget cakes, biscuits, chocolate, and any sugary foods. Eat plenty of fresh fruit and vegetables; moderate quantities of meat, fish, eggs and cheese; ½ pint/300ml fresh milk; moderate amounts of carbohydrate foods, e.g., cereal, bread, potatoes, pasta. Eat only ½oz/15g fat daily (i.e., margarine, butter, lard, cooking oil or 1oz/25g low-fat spread). Moderate your alcohol consumption. Each and every pregnant mother reacts differently to her new physical state. Some gain more than others, but there is no need whatever to pile on stones and stones through pregnancy. Take regular gentle exercise and eat well and sensibly. Avoid foods that you know are of little nutritional value, and if you feel the need to eat between meals, always have some fresh fruit handy to satisfy those hunger pangs.

Q. *Now that I am slim I only have one more wish to fulfil: I wish I could stop smoking. Everyone tells me that I am bound to gain weight. Is that true?*
A. It is a fact that if someone is a heavy smoker cigarettes can prove an effective appetite suppressant. Consequently they could find that they feel significantly more hungry when they stop. Smoking can also increase a person's

metabolic rate, which will therefore slow down when they stop.

Initially there could be a temporary weight gain caused by water retention as the body readjusts to the absence of nicotine. In the longer term weight can also creep on as a result of a combination of the following:

(a) As the nicotine is absent, the body metabolises food more efficiently and absorbs more calories and nutrients
(b) Food tastes and smells better and consequently becomes more attractive
(c) Food is a substitute for the oral pleasure that cigarettes once supplied

This all sounds rather depressing, but don't despair. Weight gain can be prevented if you adopt a patient and sensible approach to giving up smoking.

1. Start by reducing by 25 per cent the amount of cigarettes smoked each day
2. After you have conquered that first reduction, reduce the quantity still further; say down to 50 per cent of the original number
3. When you feel you can reduce that number by 50 per cent again you will be well on the way to success
4. Now try smoking only while at home or at work. Don't break your own rules
5. Try to wean yourself away from smoking by reducing the quantity smoked by one cigarette every three days
6. Then stop completely and you'll be amazed how many people are delighted! They will certainly help and encourage you

By reducing gradually the amount of nicotine you inhale over this initial six-to-eight-week period your body will have adjusted back to normal so that no weight gain should occur. So don't overeat, but do increase your physical activity. You'll be amazed how much better you will feel, so why not give it a try?

137

Q. *I've been told I must have a hysterectomy. My friends have also told me that I will inevitably gain weight and have a fat tummy. I'm so worried. Is what they say really true?*

A. No, it isn't. I had this operation six years ago. I weigh less now than I did then. I have a flat tummy and I returned to my exercise classes after six weeks. I couldn't do a lot initially, but after nine weeks I was almost back to normal. Don't sit around for weeks after your operation. Just be sensible and your body will tell you how far you can go, and if at any time your scar hurts, stop and have a rest. It is a serious operation so treat it with respect, but *don't* become lazy.

Q. *I'm frightened of overexercising because if I stop I'm sure I'll go all flabby. What should I do?*

A. Yes, you can overdo it. Just moderate your physical activity to a level where you can comfortably practise regularly without becoming a 'fitness junky'. There is no need to workout for hours every day. Four or five sensible sessions a week is what I consider to be ideal for a non-athlete.

Q. *Is it true that losing fat and building muscles can cause you to actually gain weight?*

A. Yes. Muscle tissue does weigh more than fat. This again underlines my argument against scales. You could be heavier than you think you should be for your height, but remember it is your *appearance* that is ten times more important than your weight. You could be beautifully toned all over and appear delightfully slim, so why bother with scales anyway? Scales are only useful when you are actually attempting to lose weight.

12
In conclusion

Our attitude to our weight is completely determined by our state of mind.

No one need regain their weight after losing it so magnificently. Don't look for excuses to give in. Don't become paranoid about your weight ever again.

If you do gain an inch here or there what does it matter. You are much slimmer than you used to be – don't ruin it by worrying now. You know it will go if you are sensible. If you start to 'diet' again you will almost certainly *gain* more weight, not lose it. It won't be the diet that fails – you *know* it would be *you* that breaks away from the prescribed portions. You'll be disgusted with yourself for 'failing again'. Don't start on that vicious circle.

So, forget your scales . . .
Forget about counting calories . . .
Forget about feeling hungry . . .
and forget 'bad' foods . . .

And remember, one binge is not that serious, but several could be. Please learn to be sensible. You *cannot* put back all your lost weight overnight.

Just look in the mirror and see how terrific you look. Aren't you proud of your achievement. Don't ever throw that away.

You can eat and stay slim. *I know* you can!

Other Arrow Books of interest:

THE LOW CALORIE MENU BOOK

Joyce Hughes and Audrey Eyton

On 1000 calories a day your excess weight will fairly melt away. But even the most conscientious dieter knows that 1000 calories a day can be a bit boring.

Here, at last, from *Slimming Magazine*, is a book of menus designed to give you the maximum choice and flexibility in what you eat, while carefully controlling how much. If you're tired of carrot sticks and lettuce, then what you need are

Try-Something-Different Menus * No-Fuss Menus *
Breakfast-Missers' Menus * Working Girls' Menus *
Slim-and-Sin Menus * and many more

Also included is a section on slimming tips and a handy caloric reference.

THE BEVERLY HILLS DIET

Judy Mazel

The worldwide No. 1 bestseller

At last a revolutionary diet which not only helps you shed pounds easily, but allows you to indulge in those forbidden fantasy foods — while losing weight.

Judy Mazel's diet plan, once the exclusive secret of Hollywood stars, is now available to everyone who wants to glow with energy, and have the slim trim body they always thought an impossible dream.

THE BEVERLY HILLS DIET — a unique phenomenon destined to change your life forever.

DR MANDELL'S 5-DAY ALLERGY RELIEF SYSTEM

Dr Marshall Mandell and Lynne Waller Scanlon

Do you — or anyone you know — suffer from any of the following:

compulsive eating ★ depression ★ compulsive drinking ★ hyperactivity ★ migraine ★ asthma ★ arthritis ★ chronic fatigue ★ schizophrenia ★ hypertension ★ clogged sinus ★ eczema ★ duodenal ulcers ★ multiple sclerosis ★ epilepsy.

All these and many more chronic mental, physical and psychosomatic illnesses may be the result of undiagnosed allergies. Dr Marshall Mandell's remarkable clinically-tested programme provides allergy relief in only 5 days.

COOKING FOR YOUR HEART'S CONTENT

The British Heart Foundation Cookbook

Cooking For Your Heart's Content is the first and only cookbook commissioned by the British Heart Foundation. It provides a wide variety of attractive recipes with low saturated fat content, all of which have been prepared and approved under medical supervision at Addenbrooke's Hospital, Cambridge.

'Don't learn the hard way as I did that it matters what you eat! These marvellous recipes not only look good, they taste good and do your heart no harm' *Eric Morecambe*

'This book really does give a wide selection of exceedingly mouthwatering recipes designed to make keeping on the straight and narrow, gastronomically speaking, no hardship at all' *Financial Times*

BESTSELLING NON-FICTION FROM ARROW

All these books are available from your bookshop or newsagent or you can order them direct. Just tick the titles you want and complete the form below.

☐	THE GREAT ESCAPE	Paul Brickhill	£1.75
☐	A RUMOR OF WAR	Philip Caputo	£1.95
☐	SS WEREWOLF	Charles Whiting	£1.50
☐	A LITTLE ZIT ON THE SIDE	Jasper Carrott	£1.50
☐	THE ART OF COARSE ACTING	Michael Green	£1.50
☐	THE UNLUCKIEST MAN IN THE WORLD	Mike Harding	£1.50
☐	DIARY OF A SOMEBODY	Christopher Matthew	£1.25
☐	TALES FROM A LONG ROOM	Peter Tinniswood	£1.75
☐	LOVE WITHOUT FEAR	Eustace Chesser	£1.95
☐	NO CHANGE	Wendy Cooper	£1.75
☐	MEN IN LOVE	Nancy Friday	£2.50

Postage _____

Total _____

ARROW BOOKS, BOOKSERVICE BY POST, PO BOX 29, DOUGLAS, ISLE OF MAN, BRITISH ISLES

Please enclose a cheque or postal order made out to Arrow Books Ltd for the amount due including 15p per book for postage and packing both for orders within the UK and for overseas orders.

Please print clearly

NAME ....

ADDRESS ....

....

Whilst every effort is made to keep prices down and to keep popular books in print, Arrow Books cannot guarantee that prices will be the same as those advertised here or that the books will be available.